Case Mysteries in
Pathophysiology

Second Edition

Patricia J. Neafsey, Ph.D.

University of Connecticut

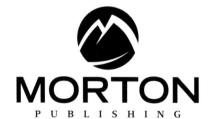

MORTON
PUBLISHING

925 W. Kenyon Avenue, Unit 12
Englewood, CO 80110

www.morton-pub.com

Book Team

Publisher: Douglas N. Morton
President: David M. Ferguson
Acquisitions Editor: Marta R. Martins
Project Manager: Melanie Stafford
Associate Project Manager: Rayna Bailey
Production Manager: Joanne Saliger
Production Assistant / Interior Design and Composition: Will Kelley
Illustrations: Imagineering Media Services, Inc.

Cover photos:
Doctors examining MRI scans, Adam Gault/ScienceSource
Blood sugar test for diabetes, VOISIN/PHANIE/ScienceSource
X-ray of fractured fibula, Scott Camazine/ScienceSource

Printed in the United States of America

10 9 8 7 6 5 4 3 2 1

ISBN-13: 978-161731-152-9

Library of Congress Control Number: 2013935086

Preface

Health science students are eager to use their knowledge of anatomy, physiology, and pathophysiology in clinical applications. The first clinical cases students encounter are likely to remain indelible in their minds because of the novelty, the interpersonal aspects, and the excitement that come with problem solving. But anatomy, physiology, and pathophysiology courses are offered during preclinical years or during early clinical rotations, when opportunities for students to care for a cardiac or renal patient may be limited. I designed *Case Mysteries in Pathophysiology* to help bridge that gap. This book offers opportunities to apply critical thinking skills to case studies while students are still in those preclinical courses.

Case Mysteries

Case Mysteries in Pathophysiology takes a problem-based learning approach. Each case presents a realistic clinical mystery—many with an interesting "twist" at the end. The case titles and associated icons are designed to help students remember details about the patient featured in each case. Normal findings (e.g., lab values, ECGs, X-rays, MRIs, CT scans, pathology slides) are presented next to the patient findings. Even though they are not expected to interpret ECGs or other images correctly at this stage of training, students will be able to identify abnormalities in these reports.

Students may work independently or with others to solve the case mysteries. They may find that working in groups is a stimulating challenge that fosters teamwork—an essential skill, as clinicians at all levels must work together to provide the best medical care possible. These case mysteries also will help students develop clinical skills in preparation for their rotations in coming years. All of the case mysteries have been revised and updated for the second edition and new case mysteries added. The illustrated answers for the cases are now available online along with web links to related content. In addition, each case has a set of multiple choice questions that can be used in a test bank or as online quizzes. We anticipate this new format will provide instructors greater flexibility in how they assess student learning.

All books evolve over time. I welcome your feedback on how this book can be improved. Contact me at **patricia.neafsey@uconn.edu**.

Disclaimer

This book was designed strictly as a learning tool for health science students. Dosages, method and duration of use, and contraindications should be verified by checking with the appropriate drug manufacturers and prescribers. The publisher and author assume no liability for injuries or harm that may take place from the application of therapies detailed in this publication.

Acknowledgments

I am especially appreciative of David Ferguson, president of Morton Publishing Company for the opportunity to publish a second edition of these case mysteries. His visionary approach to blending problem-based learning methods with superior quality visuals is a Morton hallmark. Thank you to Bernadette Madara of Southern Connecticut State University and Melanie McClure from the University of Saint Mary for their diligence in reviewing the new case mysteries and online test questions in this second edition. Their suggestions were heeded and translated to revisions of the prior cases. Editor Marta Martins and her team have been delightful to work with. Marta has a phenomenal ability to maintain a calm demeanor while managing all of the moving parts of a complex publication. Project Manager Melanie Stafford copyedited the manuscripts, and Rayna Bailey, associate project manager, pursued permissions along with Marta—tasks that require superb time management skills and dogged perseverance. Will Kelley, production assistant, produced the new text and table layout and rendered in-house illustrations—all of which give the second edition an improved visual appeal and usability. I am grateful to Carter Fenton, vice president of Sales and Marketing, without whose encouragement five years ago, this project would not have been initiated.

Many special thanks to the talented artists at Imagineering for their illustrations. I remain amazed at how well they can decipher my scribbles and capture what I see in my mind's eye. I am grateful to the more than 4,000 students who have joined me in 8 a.m. classes to explore the mysteries of pathophysiology for the past 25 years.

Finally, thank you to my family for their love, support, and patience.

Contents

The Malicious Third-Grade Cougher

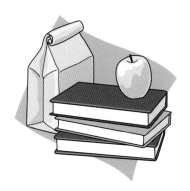

During her well-child visit in mid-September, Mary was excited to be in the third grade. "We get to read chapter books and write stories. Plus—we have a pet hamster, and we take turns taking him home. My turn is next Friday!" Mary was weighed and measured and given a physical exam. All findings were normal for an 8-year-old girl. "I sure hope we don't have a repeat of last year," her mother sighed. "I lost all my sick leave staying home with poor Mary's colds. But she's been healthy all summer—and she grew 2 inches, too!"

On October 12 Mary caught her first cold. It came and went in three days over the weekend, leaving only a dry, hacking cough. Two weeks later her teacher said to Mary's mother at a parent-teacher meeting, "I think Mary is coughing in school on purpose. She doesn't seem to cough anything up. And from what you just said, she's okay at home. I'd like to make a referral to the school psychologist."

"Give me a week," Mary's mom responded. "I want to take her back to our nurse practitioner first."

Mary's APRN asked Mary to lean over, take a deep breath, and try to cough up sputum. Mary was unable to cough up anything. The APRN listened to Mary's heart and lungs and then told her mother that she would like Mary to have an evaluation at the spirometry lab.

Mary's spirometry readings below are before and after Mary was given two puffs of a short-acting broncho-dilator called albuterol.

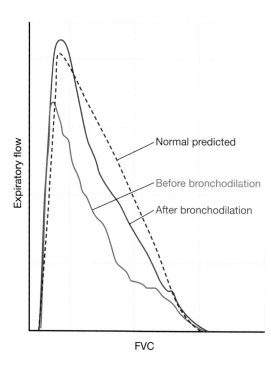

FVC

	Before Albuterol	After Albuterol	Normal (Predicted)
FEV_1	1.59 L	2.04 L	2.09 L
FVC	2.57 L	2.64 L	2.44 L
$FEV_1\%FVC$	62%	77%	86%

Sample data from: Become an Expert in Spirometry: **http://spirxpert.com**

1-1 **Mary's spirometry readings**

References

- Become an Expert in Spirometry. http://www.spirxpert.com.

- Gehle, K. 2010. *Case Studies in Environmental Medicine: Environmental Triggers of Asthma*. Washington, DC: U.S. Agency for Toxic Substances and Disease. http://www.atsdr.cdc.gov/csem/asthma/docs/asthma.pdf.

- Mayo Foundation for Medical Education and Research. *How to Use a Peak Flow Meter* (video). New York: Mayo Foundation. http://www.mayoclinic.com/health/asthma/MM00399.

- National Heart, Lung, and Blood Institute. 2007. *Guidelines for the Diagnosis and Management of Asthma*. EPR-3, July. Bethesda, MD: NHLBI. http://www.nhlbi.nih.gov/guidelines/asthma/asthgdln.pdf.

Questions

1 What is spirometry?

_____

2 What is FVC? What is FEV_1? What is $FEV_1\%FVC$? See Become an Expert in Spirometry, **http://www.spirxpert.com,** for help.

_____

_____

_____

_____

3 What do Mary's spirometry readings suggest?

_____

_____

_____

_____

_____

_____

_____

4 What problem does Mary most likely have? Why?

_____

_____

5 What is the value of a sputum culture in Mary's case?

_____

_____

6 What are the typical symptoms of this disease?

_____

_____

_____

_____

7 What are the probable triggers of Mary's cough?

8 How will Mary's cough be treated?

9 What is PEFR? How is it measured? What is it used for?

10 What other precautions should be taken for Mary?

The Uninformed Coach

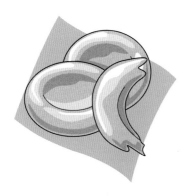

Shawn has sickle-cell disease (SCD), also known as sickle-cell anemia. He grew up knowing how serious SCD can be, but he was fortunate. He was a healthy child with no infections other than the occasional cold. His parents and brother and sister doted on him as the youngest and smallest child in the family. In high school he tried out for the track team and was able to compete in the shot put. He wasn't the best, but he was the only person who did the shot put on his team. When he went to college, it was the first time he had been away from home other than his yearly week away at the Hole in the Wall Gang Camp.

In college, Shawn liked his classes, team, and coach. It was great to be on his own! In mid-October he felt the cold while walking across campus. At first it felt good, with the fall leaves against the blue sky. By November, when he caught a common cold, he developed a pain in his left thigh. At the indoor practice the coach told him to work through it and then put a heat pack on it. "You've probably pulled a muscle from throwing the way you do. We're going to help you unlearn your bad habits. By spring you'll be able to throw twice as far."

When Shawn got back to his room, his left leg hurt more. He called his mom, who drove to the campus and took him to the emergency department. By the time he was seen, he was in so much pain that he couldn't speak. His upper abdomen hurt as much as his leg. He was having difficulty breathing.

Shown here is a photomicrograph of Shawn's blood smear.

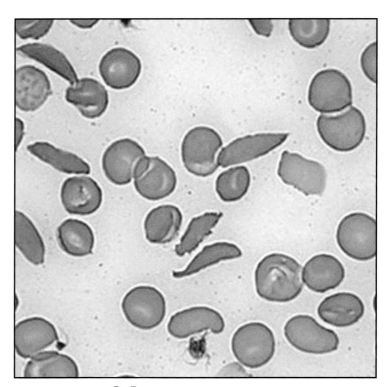

2-1 Shawn's blood smear

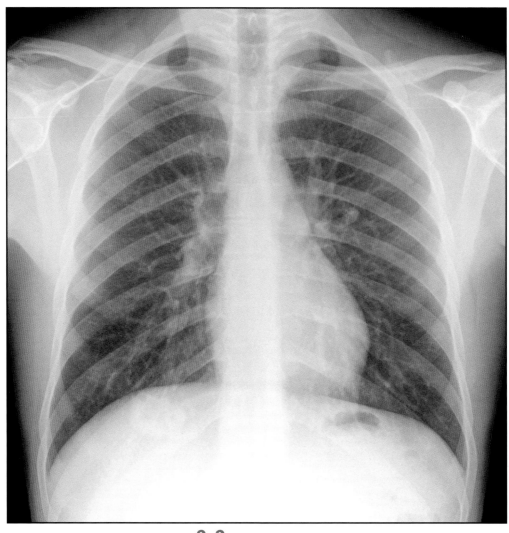

2-2 **Normal X-ray**

Shawn's X-ray is below.

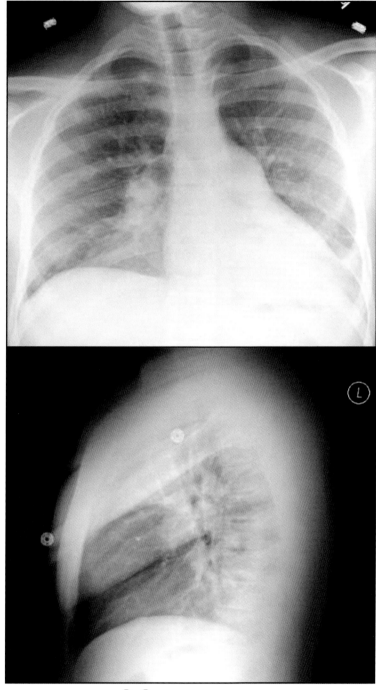

2-3 **Shawn's X-rays**

Courtesy of www.pediatriceducation.org

References

- American Sickle Cell Anemia Association. http://www.ascaa.org.

- Hole in the Wall Gang Camp. http://www.holeinthewallgang.org.

- Maakaron, J. E. 2012. "Anemia, Sickle Cell." *eMedicine* (January 3). http://emedicine.medscape.com/article/205926-overview.

- Mayo Foundation for Education and Research. *Sickle Cell Anemia*. New York: Mayo Foundation. http://www.mayoclinic.com/health/sickle-cell-anemia/DS00324.

- National Heart, Lung, and Blood Institute, Division of Blood Diseases and Resources. 2002. *The Management of Sickle Cell Disease*. Bethesda, MD: NHLBI.

Questions

1 What is the Hole in the Wall Gang Camp? See **http://www.holeinthewallgang.org** for help.

2 How is sickle-cell disease transmitted, and how common is it?

3 What happens to the red blood cell to cause sickling?

4 What are the possible complications of sickle-cell disease?

5 What acute complication of sickle-cell disease does Shawn probably have?

6 How will Shawn be treated for this complication?

Fishing Marines

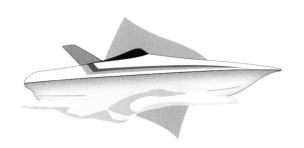

Farley Histon was now a marine. He had finished boot camp at Paris Island, was officially stationed at Camp LJ, and was going to enjoy three days of R&R on Emerald Isle. The worst part of boot camp was actually the strep throat infection he got at the end. He was now on day 7 of his cephalexin and felt fine. He and his marine buddies Jermaine and Darnell rented a motel room and reserved a charter boat to go fishing. None of them had ever gone saltwater charter fishing before—they were all from Detroit. They checked into the Dockside Motel and got on the charter boat. By 5 p.m. they were out at sea, and Jermaine caught his first king mackerel. Then, in short order, Darnell caught one. "Never have marines actually caught king mackerel on their first trip before!" shouted the captain. "I am sort of unprepared for two big ones. Stuff 'em in the cooler! We'll take a little ride down the coast so you can see the camp from the water—unless you want to keep fishin'?" "We've got the boat for three hours," said Farley. "Why not just keep fishing and see what happens?" Five minutes went by, and Farley caught a king mackerel. This one was bigger than either of the other two. "It's gotta be at least 10 pounds! Make sure I get that one when we get back!" said Farley.

When they got back to the dock, the men were tired. The thrill of getting through boot camp was finally catching up with them. Instead of building a fire on the beach and cooking some fish as they had planned, they cleaned the fish on the dock and put them in their fish cooler. They left the cooler in the motel room and then went to eat supper at the bar next door. All three were asleep by 10 p.m. The next morning, they decided to cook Farley's fish on the beach. They bought some firewood, built a firepit in the sand, and, when the coals were ready, cooked Farley's fish with some clams and corn-in-the-husk they bought at the corner market. "This is like reality TV on a tropical island," said Jermaine. "Three buff guys eating stuff they caught." "Yeah," said Farley. "You and Darnell ate food from the market. I am the only one eating the mackerel." "Well, it is your fish," said Jermaine. "We'll eat ours when we get back to camp." Farley wrapped his leftover cooked mackerel in some foil and put it in the truck for the half-hour drive back to camp.

Later that day, Farley chilled the mackerel and put it on spinach salad for his wife, Jocelyn. They both enjoyed the smoky flavor. "This was quite a good week for you, Farley! I am so proud of you!" said Jocelyn. About half an hour later, Farley told Jocelyn, "I don't feel so well. My knees are really hurting, and look how swollen they are. My head and stomach hurt, and I have heartburn. My chest is really itchy—do I have hives or something?" "Wow," said Jocelyn, "it looks like one giant hive. Can you swallow water? Maybe you are allergic to something. I am driving you right over to the navy ER." Farley's chest was bright red.

When they got to the clinic, Farley got out of the truck, and Jocelyn helped him in the door. The triage nurse took one look at him and called for a crash cart. He gave Farley a shot of epinephrine and got him on a gurney. Then he gave Farley 50 mg of Benadryl. About two hours later, Farley said his itching was a little bit better, but his knees hurt more than ever, and now his fingers were swollen. His feet had weird purple splotches on them. "Did I mess my knees and feet up in boot camp? What is going on?" he asked.

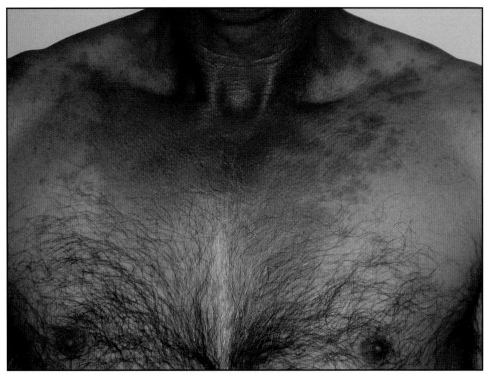

3-1 **Farley's chest**

Courtesy of DermNetNZ.org

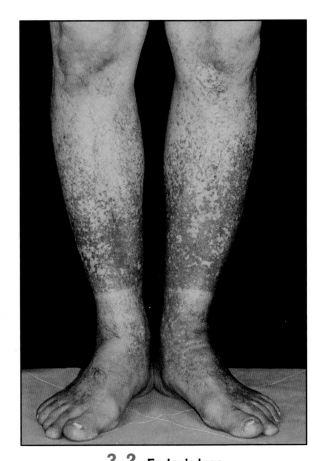

3-2 Farley's legs

Reprinted from *The Lancet* 381, no. 9862, Jui-Hung Ko and Wen-Hung Chung, "Serum Sickness," e1, 2013, with permission from Elsevier

Intake information from triage nurse:

- 23-year-old male, married

- Blood pressure: 88/54, then 111/67 at 5 minutes after 0.3 mg epinephrine IM

- Heart rate: 110, then 82 at 5 minutes after 0.3 mg epinephrine IM

- Temp: 101°F (38°C)

- History of amoxicillin allergy, age 14, taken for pharyngitis; later diagnosed as mononucleosis; developed body rash, which cleared one day after amoxicillin was discontinued

- No history of other allergies

- Patient is on day 7 of cephalexin for strep throat diagnosed from in-office quick test

- Complains of severe pruritus with headache and acute acid reflux

- Upper trunk flushed with diffuse erythematous rash, well demarcated

- Symmetrical swelling in knees and fingers

- Feet have nonblanching purpura

- Inguinal and cervical lymphadenopathy

- Negative on meningitis tests

- Lungs clear

References

- Alissa, H. M. 2011. "Serum Sickness." *eMedicine* (August 30). http://emedicine.medscape.com/article/332032-overview.

- American Geriatrics Society, Beers Criteria Update Expert Panel. 2012. "American Geriatrics Society Updated Beers Criteria for Potentially Inappropriate Medication Use in Older Adults." *Journal of the American Geriatric Society*. http://www.americangeriatrics.org/files/documents/beers/2012BeersCriteria_JAGS.pdf.

- Food Allergy and Anaphylaxis Network. http://www.foodallergy.org.

- Jagminas, L. 2012. "Percutaneous Transtracheal Jet Ventilation." *eMedicine* (June 18). http://emedicine.medscape.com/article/1413327-overview.

- Mustafa, S. S. 2012. "Anaphylaxis." *eMedicine* (February 14). http://emedicine.medscape.com/article/135065-overview.

- Noltkamper, D. 2012. "Histamine Toxicity from Fish." *eMedicine* (March 30). http://emedicine.medscape.com/article/1009464-overview.

1 What are three possible problems that could have caused Farley's symptoms?

_____

_____

_____

2 Explain the pathophysiology of each of the problems you listed above.

_____

_____

_____

_____

_____

_____

_____

_____

_____

_____

_____

_____

_____

_____

_____

_____

_____

3 What is the treatment for each of these problems?

_____

_____

_____

_____

_____

_____

_____

_____

_____

_____

_____

_____

_____

_____

_____

_____

_____

_____

4 What do you think actually caused Farley's symptoms?

_____

_____

_____

_____

_____

Suzie Feeds the Bunny

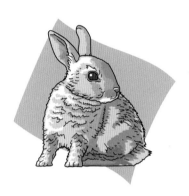

Laura invited her preschool class to her birthday party. Her pet, Bunchy Bunny, was put in his cage. Her 7-year-old brother, Jeremy, put a sign on the cage: "DO NOT FEED THE BUNNY." "That oughta do it!" He exclaimed.

"Laura," advised her mother, "make sure that none of the kids put their fingers in the cage or Bunchy might bite them, thinking they're feeding him!"

When the children arrived, the first thing Laura did was show them Bunchy.

"What does the sign say?" Suzie asked.

"Do not feed the bunny! And don't put your fingers in the cage or he will think you are food!" said Laura.

At that, Suzie immediately put her finger in the cage—and Bunchy bit her. "That hurt!" she cried, but then she ran off to see the clown who was making balloon figures.

Later that day Suzie's finger was red and swollen.

"What happened to your finger, Suzie?" her mother asked.

"I got a boo boo at Laura's party."

"How did you get the boo boo?"

"I dunno."

Suzie's mother put some triple antibiotic ointment on the wound and topped it with a bright pink bandage.

"It feels okay, Mommy," Suzie assured her.

Four weeks later Suzie's finger seemed to be healed, but her finger was still warm to the touch with local edema (swelling) and erythema (redness). She complained that she had trouble holding a crayon. "I can't move this finger like my other fingers," she said. Suzie's mother became worried and brought her to the orthopedic clinic.

An X-ray of Suzie's finger was taken, after which she immediately was given a magnetic resonance image (MRI) of her legs and arms. An MRI is a diagnostic imaging technique whereby the patient is placed in a strong, uniform magnetic field. Protons absorb energy from the magnetic field and then emit radio waves as their excitation decays. These radio frequency signals are converted into three-dimensional images. MRIs do not expose patients to ionizing radiation.

Below is an X-ray of Suzie's finger:

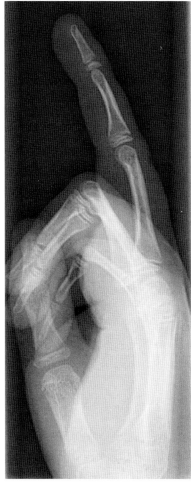

Courtesy of Sarah J. Fitch,
Virginia Commonwealth University,
Department of Pathology

4-1 X-ray of Suzie's finger

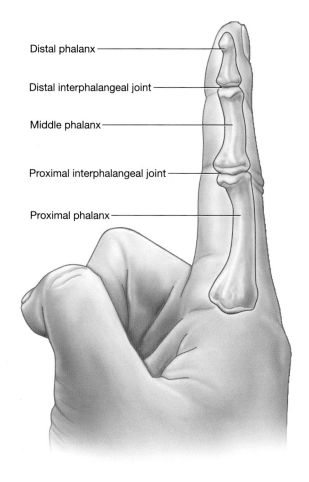

Distal phalanx

Distal interphalangeal joint

Middle phalanx

Proximal interphalangeal joint

Proximal phalanx

4-2 Anatomy of finger

References

- King, R. W. 2011. "Osteomyelitis in Emergency Medicine." *eMedicine* (July 27). http://emedicine.medscape.com/article/785020-overview.

- Latham, E. 2012. "Hyperbaric Oxygen Therapy." *eMedicine* (May 24). http://emedicine.medscape.com/article/1464149-overview.

1 Find the dorsal aspect of the metaphysis of the distal phalanx on the X-ray. What do you see?

_____

_____

2 What condition does Suzie have?

_____

_____

_____

_____

3 Where else can this condition occur in the body?

_____

_____

_____

_____

_____

_____

4 How could this problem have been prevented?

_____

_____

_____

5 What could happen if this problem is not treated?

_____

_____

_____

_____

_____

6 Why was Suzie given an MRI of her legs and arms?

_____

_____

_____

_____

_____

7 What else can cause this problem?

_____

_____

_____

_____

8 How can this problem be treated?

_____

_____

_____

_____

_____

_____

_____

_____

_____

_____

_____

_____

_____

_____

_____

_____

Favorite Uncle

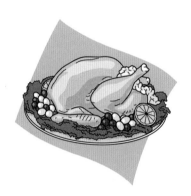

Uncle Jed, the family's favorite uncle, choked on a turkey bone in his soup three days after Thanksgiving. He was able to cough up the little bone, but he began to hemorrhage from the esophagus. He was rushed to the emergency department, where he was intubated, and a rapid infusion of 5% dextrose plus thiamine and colloid solution was started. He also was given an infusion of Sandostatin (octreotide acetate) to stop the bleeding. His blood was typed, and he received fresh frozen plasma, fresh blood, and vitamin K1. He received endoscopic variceal ligation, in which elastic bands were placed around two ruptured varices (varicose veins) to strangle and obliterate them. He will require this procedure every two to three weeks until the esophageal varices have disappeared. He has been started on a beta blocker propranolol 40 mg PO bid and an ethanol drip. He has a nasogastric tube and is NPO for the next 24 hours. Gastric lavage through the nasogastric tube will be performed repeatedly over the next 24 hours to examine aspirated stomach contents and identify any rebleeding.

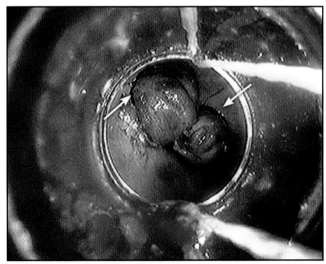

5-1 **Screening for esophageal varices**

Reproduced with permission from J.S. Goff, "Endoscopic Variceal Ligation."
In: *UpToDate*, Basow, D.S. (ed.), UpToDate, Waltham, MA 2013. Copyright ©2013
UpToDate, Inc. For more information visit www.uptodate.com.

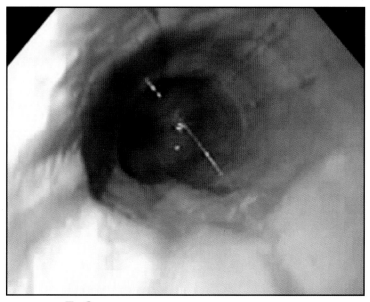

5-2 **Endoscope of normal esophagus**

Courtesy of Medical College of Wisconsin

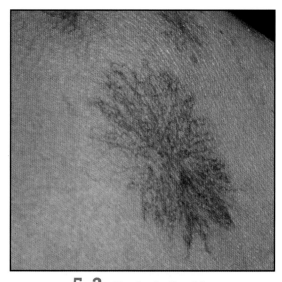

5-3 **Uncle Jed's skin**

Herbert L. Fred, MD, and Hendrik A. van Dijk,
Images of Memorable Cases—50 Years at the Bedside
(Houston: Long Tail Press/Rice University Press, 2007)

Uncle Jed's niece Janice and nephew Greg just visited him. "Whoa!" said Greg. "Uncle Jed has man-boobs! But otherwise he looks okay. He does have a great tan."

"I don't know about that tan," Janice responded. "It looks pretty orange—probably fake! But he does have breasts—and stretch marks on his beer belly. Weird. Did you notice that he also has no hair on his arms or legs? He seems to have changed since last Thanksgiving—not just the tan thing either. He has red splotches on his nose and cheeks, and his palms are really red. But the thing I worry about the most is that he seems to lie about things. And not in a kidding way like when we were kids. I asked him which kennel his dog was in so I could call and tell them to keep Snarl another week. And Uncle Jed told me that Snarl was at home with Aunt Sally. Well, Aunt Sally died of breast cancer two years ago. Does Uncle Jed have Alzheimer's disease?"

Following are selected lab values from Uncle Jed, 24 hours after admission.

Test	Value	SI Units	Reference Range	SI Units
Ammonia	97 mcg/dL	57 µmol/L	19–60 mcg/dL	11–35 µmol/L
BUN	42 mg/dL	15 mmol/L	7–18 mg/dL	2.5–6.9 mmol/L
Creatinine, serum	1.52 mg/dL	134 µmol/L	0.8–1.3 mg/dL	71–115 µmol/L
Bilirubin, total	1.7 mg/dL	29 µmol/L	0.1–1.0 mg/dL	1.7–17.1 µmol/L
Bilirubin, direct (conjugated)	0.3 mg/dL	5.1 µmol/L	0.1–0.3 mg/dL	1.7–5.1 µmol/L
Bilirubin, indirect (unconjugated)	1.4 mg/dL	24 µmol/L	0.2–0.8 mg/dL	3.4–13.7 µmol/L
Protein, total	5.5 g/dL	55 g/L	6.4–8.2 g/dL	64–82 g/L
Albumin	2.4 g/L	24 g/L	3.4–5.0 g/dL	34–50 g/L
Alkaline phosphatase	157 U/L		50–136 U/L	
Aspartate aminotransferase/ SGOT (AST/SGOT)	49 U/L		15–37 U/L	
Alanine aminotransferase/ SGOT (ALT/SGOT)	71 U/L		30–65 U/L	
Gamma-glutamyl transferase (GGT)	139		1–94 U/L	
Cholesterol, total	230 mg/dL	5.9 mmol/L	50–199 mg/dL	1.3–5.2 mmol/L
Triglycerides	301 mg/dL	3.4 mmol/L	15–149 mg/dL	0.17–1.7 mmol/L
RBC	4.1		4.50–5.90 K/cmm	
Hemoglobin (HGB)	13.5 g/dL	135 g/L	13.5–17.5 g/dL	135–175 g/L
Hematocrit (HCT)	37%		41.0–53.0%	
Mean Corpuscular volume (MCV)	102 fL		80–100 fL	
Mean corpuscular hemoglobin (MCH)	26 pg		26.0–34.0 pg	
Mean corpuscular hemoglobin concentration (MCHC)	31.0 g/dL	310 g/L	31.0–37.0 g/dL	310–370 g/L
Prothrombin time (PT)	14 seconds		9–12 seconds	

References

- Azer, A. 2010. "Esophageal Varices." *eMedicine* (May 19). http://www.eMedicine.com/med/topic745.htm.

- O'Shea, R. S., S. Dasarathy, A. J. McCullough, and the Practice Guideline Committee of the American Association for the Study of Liver Diseases and the Practice Parameters Committee of the American College of Gastroenterology. 2010. "Alcoholic Liver Disease." *Hepatology* 51, no. 1: 308–328. http://www.aasld.org/practiceguidelines/Documents/Bookmarked%20Practice%20Guidelines/AlcoholicLiverDisease1-2010.pdf.

- "Standard Drink Conversion." http://www.virginia.edu/case/ATOD/standard-drink-conversion.html.

1 What health problem does Uncle Jed probably have?

_____

_____

2 What caused the esophageal varices?

_____

_____

_____

_____

_____

3 Why would Uncle Jed be started on a beta blocker (which slows the heart and lowers blood pressure)?

_____

_____

4 Why would Uncle Jed be started on an ethanol drip?

_____

_____

_____

_____

_____

_____

_____

5 Why was Uncle Jed given thiamine along with the dextrose infusion?

_____

_____

_____

_____

6 Why does Uncle Jed have breasts, stretch marks, a tan, and red marks on his face?

7 Uncle Jed is positive for hepatitis C. How does this viral infection play a part in his current problem and prognosis?

8 What other problems might Uncle Jed have?

9 Why is Uncle Jed telling lies?

_____

_____

_____

10 What is Uncle Jed's prognosis? Are there any treatments for this?

_____

_____

_____

_____

_____

_____

_____

_____

_____

_____

_____

_____

_____

_____

_____

_____

_____

The Red Hat Hikers

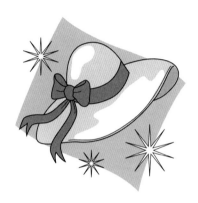

The Red Hat Hikers, a group of 60-something-year-old women, meet once a week to hike Mt. Monadnock, the second-most climbed mountain in the world after Mt. Fuji. On the schedule this week was the Pumpelly Trail, an arduous four-hour climb with several hand-and-foot "scrambles" and a long view of the looming peak. All were ready with their hiking poles and camelback water bags. Sue was snack leader: "This week it's chocolate-covered dried cranberries, girls!"

"What—no gorp this week?" exclaimed the other four women. (Gorp, referring to trail mix, is an acronym for "good 'ole raisins and peanuts," but it often includes chocolate chips.)

"Nope—these little things are supposed to be good for the bladder, and we can all use a little help there!"

The group soon settled into a stride where they could keep up a conversation in the humid 88 degree weather. When they got to the top, it was definitely a "summit day"—clear and cool, around 70 degrees. They munched their snack, drank water, and after about a 45-minute rest, started down the way they came, with fabulous views of the fall foliage to the north. As they descended, the air temperature got warmer and more humid.

"Temperature inversion!" Nan announced, "when the dense, cold air at the top traps the warm humid air at the bottom."

Sue had consumed all of her water from her hydration pack and gasped. "Whoa—I just saw something weird, like a mountain lion, only it looked like a calico cat."

"Right," the others said, amused.

When the group reached the end of the bare rock above tree line, just before the last steep descent, Sue fell over backward.

"What's wrong, Sue?" Nan quickly asked.

"I feel like my brain is shutting down. I can't find my words. Is this a side effect from my SSRI?" Sue's voice trailed off.

Nan dialed 911, and a rescue team arrived in fewer than 15 minutes. The medics put Sue on a mountain gurney and brought her down to a waiting ambulance.

Selected lab values from Sue's admission to the emergency department are as follows:

Test	Value (nonfasting)	SI Units	Reference/Range	SI Units
Sue's Lab Values				
Glucose	115 mg/dL	6.38 mmol/L	< 200 mg/dL	< 11.1 mmol/L
BUN	8 mg/dL	2.8 mmol/L	7–18 mg/dL	2.5–6.4 mmol/L
Creatinine, serum	0.9 mg/dL	79 µmol/L	0.8–1.3 mg/dL	71–115 µmol/L
Bilirubin, total	0.2 mg/dL	3.4µmol/L	0.1–1.0 mg/dL	1.71–17.1 µmol/L
Protein, total	6.5 g/dL	65 g/L	6.4–8.2 g/dL	64–82 g/L
Albumin	3.4 g/dL	44 g/L	3.4–5.0 g/dL	34–50 g/L
Alkaline phosphatase	130 U/L		50–136 U/L	
AST/SGOT	29 U/L		15–37 U/L	
ALT/SGOT	41 U/L		30–65 U/L	
GGT	39 U/L		1–94 U/L	
Cholesterol, total	180 mg/dL	4.6 mmol/L	50–199 mg/dL	1.3–5.1 mmol/L
Triglycerides	75 mg/dL	0.85 mmol/L	15–149 mg/dL	0.17–1.7 mmol/L
WBC	5.1 K/cmm		4.5–11.0 K/cmm	
RBC	4.0 K/cmm		4.00–5.20 K/cmm	
HGB	11.9 g/dL	119 g/L	12.0–16.0 g/dL	120–160 g/L
HCT	35.8%		36.0–46.0%	
MCV	90 fL		80–100 fL	
MCH	31.2 pg		26.0–34.0 pg	
MCHC	33.7 g/dL	337 g/L	31.0–37.0 g/dL	310–370 g/L
PT (prothrombin time)	11 seconds		9–12 seconds	
Sodium	129 mEq/L	129 mmol/L	136–145 mEq/L	136–145 mmol/L
Potassium	4.5 mEq/L	4.5 mmol/L	3.5–5.1 mEq/L	3.5–5.1 mmol/L
Chloride	97 mEq/L	97 mmol/L	98–107 mEq/L	98–107 mmol/L
CO_2, Total	26.3 mEq/L	26.3 mmol/L	21.0–32.0 mEq/L	21.0–32.0 mmol/L
Anion gap	10.7 mEq/L	10.7 mmol/L	8.0–17.0 mEq/L	8.0–17.0 mmol/L
Calcium	8.5 mg/dL	2.1 mmol/L	8.5–10.5 mg/dL	2.1–2.6 mmol/L

References

- Cycling Performance Tips. "Risks of Overhydration with Exercise." http://www.cptips.com/water.htm.

- Iowa State University Extension to Families. "Fluids." http://www.extension.iastate.edu/families/fluids.

- Luzzio, C. L. 2011. "Central Pontin Myelinolysis." *Medscape Reference.* http://emedicine.medscape.com/article/1174329-overview.

- Murray, B., J. Stofann, and E. R. Eichner. 2003. "Hyponatremia in Athletes." *Sports Science Exchange* 88, no. 16. http://www.gssiweb.com/Article_Detail.aspx?articleID=604.

- Neafsey, P. J. 2004. "Thiazides and Selective Serotonin Reuptake Inhibitors Can Induce Hyponatremia." *Home Healthcare Nurse* 22, no. 11: 788–790.

Questions

1 Which lab values are abnormal?

_____

_____

2 What problem does Sue have?

_____

_____

_____

3 What is the most likely cause of this problem?

_____

_____

_____

_____

_____

_____

4 What are physical symptoms of this problem?

_____

_____

5 How could this problem have been prevented?

_____

_____

_____

6 How can this problem be treated?

_____

_____

_____

_____

_____

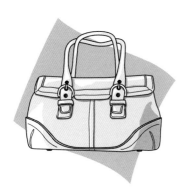

Grandma's Got a Brand-New Bag

Luanne Lin, age 83, was brought into the emergency department with upper gastrointestinal bleeding. She said she did not have any pain, but "all of a sudden I coughed and then I started to choke up bright red blood." By the time she reached the hospital, the bleeding had stopped. Her blood test results showed no abnormalities in coagulation. Her red blood cell (RBC) count was 3.5 K/cmm (normal: 4.00–5.20 K/cmm), but all other values were in the normal range. Her blood pressure was 110/70 mm Hg supine and 100/60 mm Hg standing. In Ms. Lin's purse was a pack of cigarettes, and in her wallet was a list of her prescription medications:

- spironolactone/HCTZ, 25 mg/25 mg: Take in a.m. for hypertension
- sertraline (generic Zoloft), 25 mg: Take in a.m. for depression
- OTC nicotinic acid, 50 mg: Take in p.m. for high triglycerides

"The other pills I take are in a bag that my daughter is bringing in. I can't remember just now what else I take—I feel so lightheaded!"

Ms. Lin was given an IV infusion of normal saline. She was prepared for an endoscopic exam of her esophagus, stomach, and duodenum—an upper GI. A topical anesthetic was sprayed into the back of her throat, and she was given an IV sedative (propofol) to relax her and suppress her gag reflex. The gastroenterologist then threaded the endoscope (a thin, flexible plastic tube equipped with a miniature camera) into Ms. Lin's mouth, down her esophagus to her stomach and duodenum.

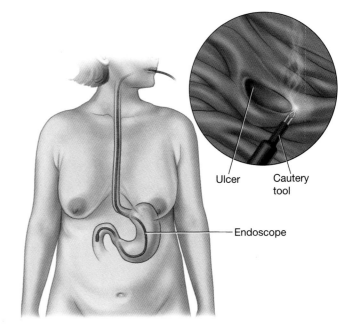

Ulcer Cautery tool

Endoscope

7-1 Endoscope of upper GI

Below is a photograph of the only abnormality seen with the endoscope. Because there was no active bleeding or clot, the area was not treated. A biopsy sample was removed for further analysis.

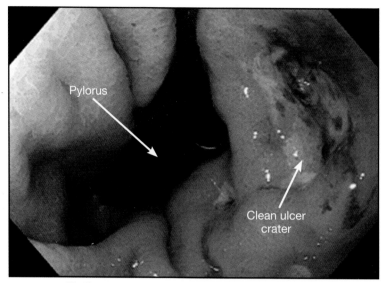

7-2 **Abnormality in Ms. Lin's endoscope**

Courtesy of the American College of Gastroenterology

A photomicrograph of the gastric biopsy specimen under high power shows inflammation and gram negative bacteria.

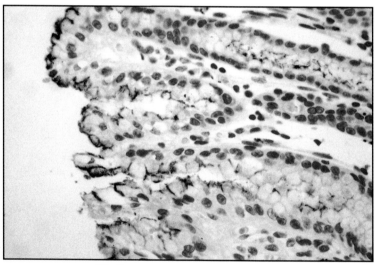

7-3 **Ms. Lin's gastric biopsy**

Courtesy of Abcam, Inc. Copyright 2013 Abcam, Inc.

References

- Anand, B. S. 2012. "Peptic Ulcer Disease." *eMedicine* (June 7). http://emedicine.medscape.com/article/181753-overview.

- Cerulli, M. 2011. "Upper Gastrointestinal Bleeding." *eMedicine* (November 25). http://emedicine.medscape.com/article/187857-overview.

- Santacroce, L., and G. Miragliotta. 2011. "*Helicobacter Pylori* Infection." *eMedicine* (September 22). http://emedicine.medscape.com/article/176938-overview.

- Vega, C. P. 2012. "Better Treatment for *Helicobacter Pylori*? A Best Evidence Review." *Medscape Family Medicine* (November 5). http://www.medscape.com/viewprogram/8097_pnt.

1 Why was Ms. Lin given an IV infusion of normal saline?

2 What problem does Ms. Lin have?

3 What is the cause of Ms. Lin's problem?

4 What medications and self-medication behaviors can cause/aggravate her problem?

5 How will Ms. Lin's problem be treated?

Sisters for Life

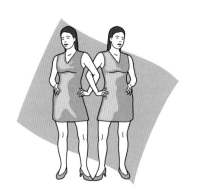

Mary and Susan Madison are 30-year-old twin sisters who were adopted at age 2. They had a double wedding, and their families live in the same duplex. They even go to medical appointments together. At today's ob/gyn appointment, Susan's blood pressure is normal at 115/70. Her urine is normal. Susan's only complaint is that she has a chronic, intermittent headache in her right temple that she thinks is a migraine. Nothing much helps the headache, but if she relaxes, the pain usually goes away on its own.

Mary's blood pressure is 165/96. Blood (hematuria) and protein (albuminuria) are found in her urine. Mary reports that she has gained about 15 pounds in the past year and has developed lower back pain and stomach pain that can be relieved by acetaminophen (for example, Tylenol). The ob/gyn notes that Mary appears to have less muscle mass in her arms and legs and less subcutaneous fat than Susan does. Mary is prescribed an antibiotic for a suspected urinary tract infection, and her urine sample is cultured for confirmation. (Later that week the culture report comes back indicating that Mary did have a urinary tract infection.)

Mary's ob/gyn uses an ultrasound to examine her back and abdomen. Both of Mary's kidneys are about four times larger than normal and appear to contain numerous fluid-filled cysts. Without further examining Susan, the ob/gyn refers *both* sisters to a nephrologist for magnetic resonance images (MRIs) of their kidneys.

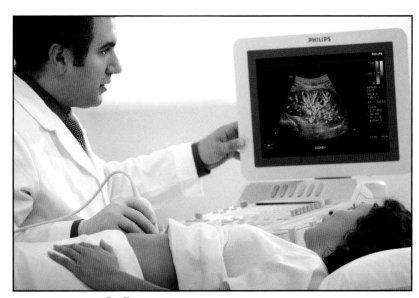

8-1 **Ultrasound exam of abdomen**

Below are the MRI images of Susan's and Mary's kidneys.

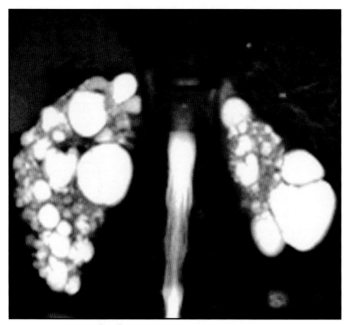

8-2 Susan's kidney MRI

Courtesy of Kyongtae Bae, MD, PhD, MR imaging radiologist whose
research on imaging PKD has been supported by the NIDDK

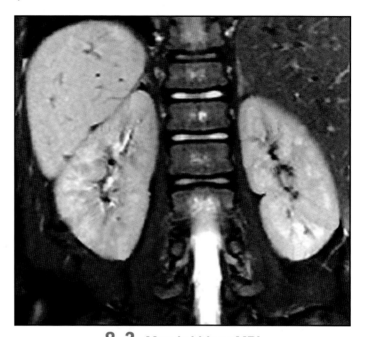

8-3 Mary's kidney MRI

Courtesy of Carol and James Herscot Center for Tuberous
Sclerosis Complex and www.massgeneral.org./livingwithtsc

The nephrologist sends both sisters to have an MRI of the brain and an echocardiogram of the heart. An MRI is a diagnostic imaging technique whereby the patient is put in a strong, uniform magnetic field. Protons absorb energy from the magnetic field and then emit radio waves as their excitation decays. These radio frequency signals are converted into three-dimensional images. MRIs do not expose patients to ionizing radiation. An echocardiogram is a series of images of the heart obtained from the reflection or transmission of ultrasonic waves through cardiac tissue.

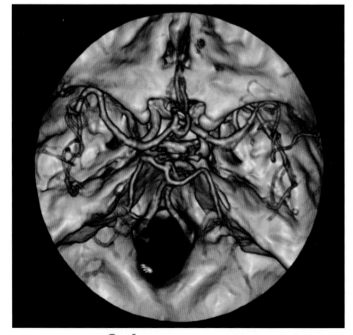

8-4 Mary's brain MRI

Courtesy of Hitachi Medical Systems, Europe Holding AG

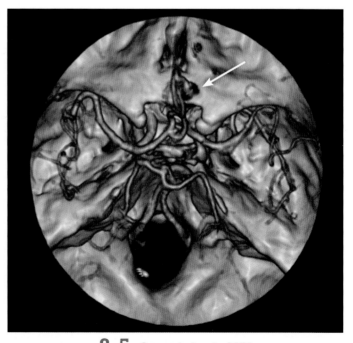

8-5 Susan's brain MRI

Courtesy of Hitachi Medical Systems, Europe Holding AG

Mary's brain MRI is normal, but Susan's is not. Susan undergoes a cerebral angiogram. A cerebral angiogram involves inserting a catheter into the femoral artery and moving it to the carotid artery. A radio opaque contrast material then is injected. The contrast material blocks the passage of X-rays and allows visualization of blood vessels in the brain on a fluoroscope (an X-ray machine that projects images on a television monitor). Mary's MRI scan is below, left. Susan's MRI scan is below, right.

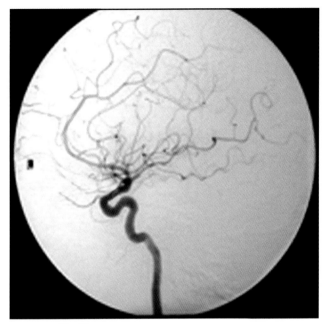

8-6 **Normal cerebral angiogram**

Courtesy of Ched Nwagwu, MD

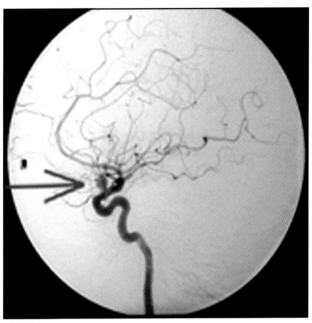

8-7 **Susan's cerebral angiogram** The arrow points to an out-pouching on the cerebral artery.

Courtesy of Ched Nwagwu, MD

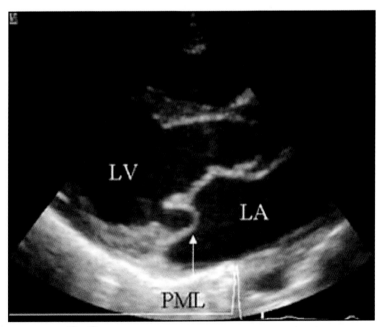

8-8 **Susan's echocardiogram showing a prolapsed mitral valve**

Reproduced with permission of the Cleveland Clinic Center for Continuing Education. R.J. Curtin and B.P. Griffin, "Mitral Valve Disease: Stenosis and Regurgitation." Disease Management Project (http://www.clevelandclinicmeded.com/medicalpubs/diseasemanagement/cardiology/mitral-valve-disease).

References

- American Dental Association. "Antibiotic Prophylaxis." http://www.ada.org/2157.aspx.

- National Institute of Neurological Disorders and Stroke. "Cerebral Aneurysm Fact Sheet." http://www.ninds.nih.gov/disorders/cerebral_aneurysm/detail_cerebral_aneurysms.htm.

- National Kidney and Urologic Diseases Information Clearinghouse. http://kidney.niddk.nih.gov/kudiseases/pubs/polycystic.

- PKD Foundation. http://www.pkdcure.org.

1 What problem does Mary have, what causes it, and how common is it? See **http://www.pkdcure.org** for help.

_____

_____

2 Why did the ob/gyn send *both* sisters for MRIs of their kidneys?

_____

_____

_____

3 What did the kidney MRIs suggest about Mary? About Susan?

_____

_____

_____

_____

_____

4 Why did Mary gain 15 pounds during the past year?

_____

_____

5 Why does Mary have high blood pressure and a urinary tract infection?

_____

_____

_____

_____

_____

_____

6 | Why did the nephrologist send both sisters for a cerebral angiogram and an echocardiogram?

7 | Would Susan be a good candidate to give one of her kidneys to Mary?

Andie's Tavern

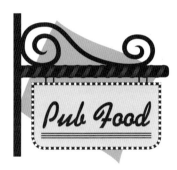

Maggie Symes, age 52, inherited Andie's Tavern from her father 30 years ago. The bar and grill has been in Maggie's family in Anderson since 1870. Maggie and her husband, Mac, managed the tavern together until Mac died of a heart attack two years ago. In addition to running Andie's, Maggie also takes care of her 4-year-old twin granddaughters during the day when the tavern is closed while her daughter works as an aide (CNA) on the 7 a.m. to 3 p.m. shift at the local nursing home. The twins have just gone back to preschool after being home for a week with colds. Maggie caught the cold and now has a fever and a productive cough. She is in the walk-in clinic and hopes to get a prescription and be on her way in time to pick up the girls from preschool. She calls her daughter, who says, "Mom, it's good to get there early this time; remember you had two bouts with bronchitis last winter when the girls brought home colds! It seems like you just never really get over them. And you seem to always be out of breath—even walking in the grocery store!"

The following information is collected at Maggie's visit:

- Female, age 52. Widow.
- Height: 5'5" (165 cm)
- Weight: 148 lbs. (67.3 kg)
- Tavern owner, caregiver for 4-year-old twin granddaughters
- Nonsmoker (last smoked at age 18)
- Nondrinker
- No use of prescription medications

- Uses acetaminophen for pain, fever
- Temperature (ear): 102°F (38.9°C)
- Pulse: 92
- Blood pressure: 139/86
- Productive cough with green sputum
- Dyspnea when walking
- Clubbed index fingers
- Two prior diagnoses of bronchitis in previous year

A photograph of Maggie Symes's index fingers is below, right.

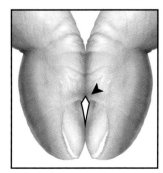

9-1 Normal index fingers

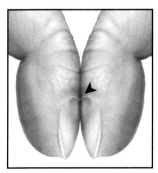

9-2 Maggie Symes's index fingers

When the nurse practitioner sees the reading as pulse: 86, SpO_2: 88% (normal is 95–100%), she sends Maggie Symes down the hall for a spirometry evaluation. After Maggie inhales albuterol (a $beta_2$ agonist bronchodilator), she is given the spirometry tests. Maggie's spirometry results are as follows. Maggie's volume of air forcibly exhaled from the point of maximum inspiration (forced vital capacity, or FVC) and her volume of air exhaled during the first second (forced expiratory volume in 1 second, FEV_1) are measured. See Become an Expert in Spirometry, **http://www.spirxpert.com**.

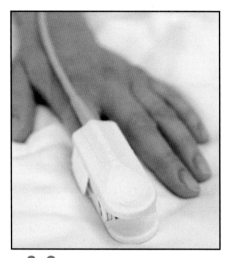

9-3 **Using a pulse oximeter**

Courtesy of Shuttershock

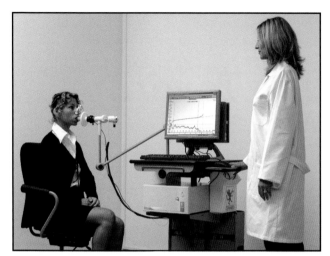

9-4 **Using a spirometer**

Courtesy of Cosmed

Maggie's Test Results

	Pre-Albuterol	Post-Albuterol	Normal (Predicted)	Post-Albuterol % Predicted
FEV_1	1.43 L	1.59 L	2.7 L	58.9%
FVC	2.42 L	2.57 L	3.4 L	75.6%
FEV_1/FVC	.59	.61	> .70	

References

- Become an Expert in Spirometry. http://www.spirxpert.com.

- Centers for Disease Control. "Chronic Obstructive Pulmonary Disease (COPD)." http://www.cdc.com.

- Centers for Disease Control. "Smoke-free Policies Improve Health." http://www.cdc.gov/tobacco/data_statistics/fact_sheets/secondhand_smoke/protection/improve_health/index.htm

- Eisner, M. D., A. K. Smith, and P. D. Blanc. 1998. "Bartenders' Respiratory Health after Establishment of Smoke-free Bars and Taverns." *Journal of the American Medical Association* 280, no. 22: 1909–1914.

- Global Initiative for Chronic Obstructive Lung Disease (GOLD). 2011. *Global Strategy for Diagnosis, Management, and Prevention of COPD.* http://www.goldcopd.org.

- Learn About COPD, http://www.learnaboutcopd.org.

- National Academy of Sciences, Institute of Medicine. 2009. "Secondhand Smoke Exposure and Cardiovascular Effects: Making Sense of the Evidence." http://www.iom.edu/Reports/2009/Secondhand-Smoke-Exposure-and-Cardiovascular-Effects-Making-Sense-of-the-Evidence/Report-Brief-Secondhand-Smoke.aspx.

- Public Health Agency of Canada. "Chronic Obstructive Pulmonary Disease." http://www.phac-aspc.gc.ca/index-eng.php.

1 What problem do you think Maggie Symes has? What information from her presenting data leads you to this conclusion?

_____

_____

_____

_____

_____

2 What are the risk factors for this problem? Which risk factors does Maggie have?

_____

_____

_____

_____

_____

_____

_____

_____

3 Describe the pathophysiology of this problem in Maggie Symes's case.

_____

_____

_____

_____

_____

_____

4   How common is this problem in North America and globally? What are the long-term consequences if it is not diagnosed early and treated? See **http://www.cdc.gov** and **http://phac-aspc.gc.ca/index-eng.php** for help.

5   What other types of this problem are there, and how does the pathophysiology differ from what Maggie is experiencing?

6 What is a pulse oximeter, and how does it work? What factors can affect pulse oximeter values?

7 How severe is Maggie Symes's problem? See **http://www.goldcopd.org** for help.

8 How will Maggie Symes's problem be managed?

9 What states/counties/towns still allow smoking in bars and taverns? What is the evidence for improved health of workers following smoking bans in restaurants and bars? See **http://www.stateoftobaccocontrol.org** for help.

The Perfect Diet

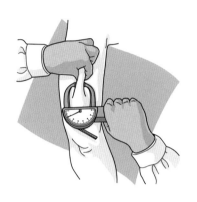

haron Rock, age 21, is hospitalized with severe abdominal pain. The pain is a "10" on a 0–10 pain scale but is intermittent. She vomits after each pain wave. Her abdomen is distended and measures 38 inches (97 cm). A clinical dietitian measures her mid-arm circumference and triceps skinfold thickness. She is given a pregnancy test. A flat-plate X-ray of her abdomen shows air under the diaphragm. Another X-ray shows a "density" (an area that blocks the X-rays) in her duodenum. She has tachypnea (rapid breathing) and dyspnea (difficulty breathing). When a stethoscope is placed over her lower abdomen, there are no bowel sounds.

Here are some of Sharon's test results:

- Height: 5'5" (165 cm)
- Weight: 100 lbs. (45 kg)
- Pregnancy test: Negative

Sharon's Test Results

Test	Value	SI Units	Reference Values	SI Units
Mid-arm circumference	18 cm		28.5 cm	
Triceps skinfold	8 mm		16.5 mm	
Potassium	5.2 mEq/L	5.2 mmol/L	3.5–5.0 mEq/L	3.5–5.0 mmol/L
Albumin	3.0 g/L	30 g/L	4.0–5.5 g/dL	40–55 g/L

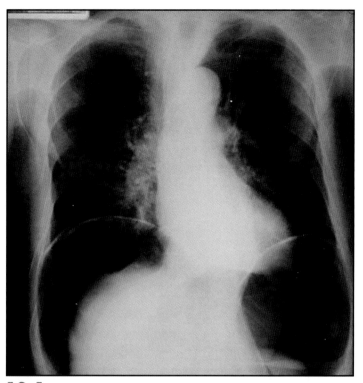

10-1 X-ray showing air under the diaphragm

Courtesy of McGill Molson Medical Informatics Project

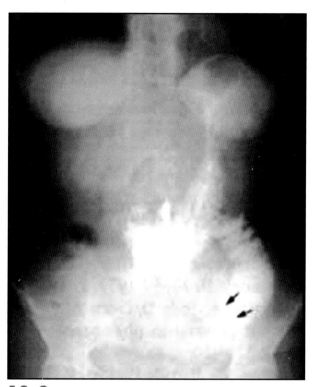

10-2 X-ray showing density in small intestine

Courtesy of the Medical University
of South Carolina's Digestive Disease Center

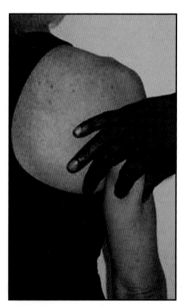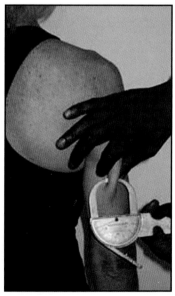

10-3 Measurement of triceps skinfold

Courtesy of Beta Technology

References

■ Kidney.org. "Methods for Performing Anthropometry and Calculating Body Measurements and Reference Tables." http://www.kidney.org/ professionals/kdoqi/guidelines_updates/nut_ appx07a.html.

■ Lange Service Center. "Using the Lange Skinfold Caliper." http://www.langeservicecenter.com/ Lange%20Manual.pdf.

Questions

1 What do the mid-arm circumference and triceps skinfold results suggest? See **http://www.kidney.org/ professionals/kdoqi/guidelines_updates/nut_appx07a.html** for help. Use the following equation for mid-arm muscle circumference (MAMC) using her mid-arm circumference (MAC) and triceps skinfold (TSF) values (normal: 23.2):

$$MAMC = MAC \text{ (cm)} - (3.14 \times TSF \text{ (cm)})$$

Draw a diagram showing a cross section of an arm with these measurements.

2 What do the X-rays suggest?

3 Why is her abdomen distended? (Give two reasons!)

4 Why is her potassium high?

5 Why does she have tachypnea and dyspnea?

6 Sharon is brought in for emergency surgery. What do you expect the surgeon will find?

The Casino Bus

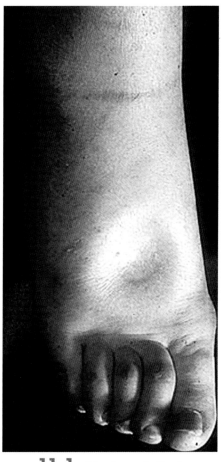

CASE 11

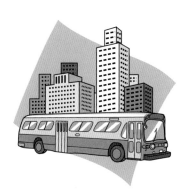

Mr. Jones, age 77, is a retired middle school history teacher. He has just been admitted as the first patient in the new hospital wing, paid for in part by two nearby casinos. Mr. Jones took the casino bus from his home, three hours away. He took a Benadryl so he could "sleep on the bus." After "playing the slots" for only 20 minutes, he began to have difficulty breathing. Someone called 911, and Mr. Jones was brought to the emergency department.

He reports that he has had "heart failure" and "COPD" but did not bring any medications or a list of his medications with him. His dyspnea responded to oxygen, an inhaled β_2 agonist (albuterol), and inhaled Atrovent (ipratropium bromide), a short-acting anticholinergic drug. His arterial blood gas values (ABGs) on admission are as follows:

Mr. Jones' Lab Values		
Test	**Value**	**Normal Range**
PaO_2	55 mm Hg	75–100 mm Hg
SaO_2	88%	94%–98%
$PaCO_2$	46 mm Hg	35–45 mm Hg
PH	7.3	7.35–7.45
HCO_3	30	22–26 mEq/L

He has + 4 pedal edema, sometimes called "pitting edema." Shown here is a photograph of his foot.

11-1 **Mr. Jones's foot**

Courtesy of the Department of Pathology, Virginia Commonwealth University, and the VCU Health System

His ECG, shown below, suggests he may have left ventricular hypertrophy (LVH). His QRS duration is more than 90 milliseconds, and he has a nonspecific T-wave abnormality. His PR interval is prolonged at 200 ms. He has a greater QRS amplitude; note the tall R waves in the left-sided leads (I, aVL, V5, V6) and the deep S waves in the right-sided leads (III, aVR, V1–V3). Although his ECG satisfies the voltage criteria for left ventricular hypertrophy, only an echocardiogram can confirm LVH. Some individuals with LVH have normal ECGs. (See http://lifeinthefastlane.com/ecg-library/basics/left-ventricular-hypertrophy.)

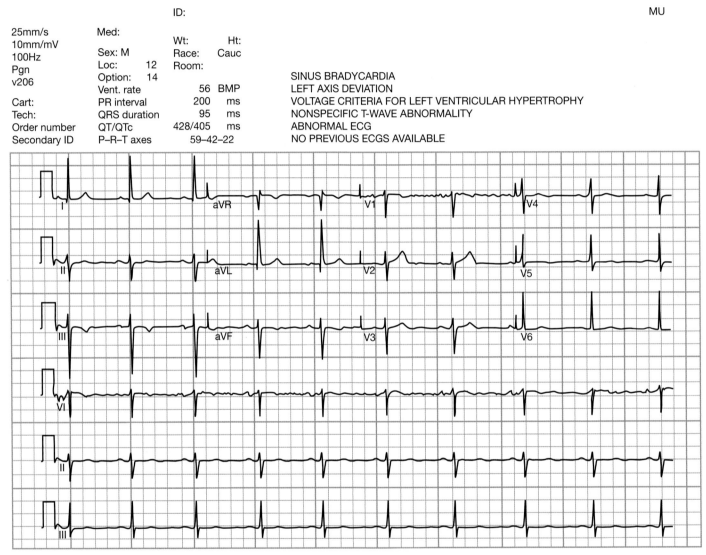

11-2 **Mr. Jones's ECG**

Courtesy of Edward Vandenberg, University of Nebraska Medical Center

A normal ECG is shown below.

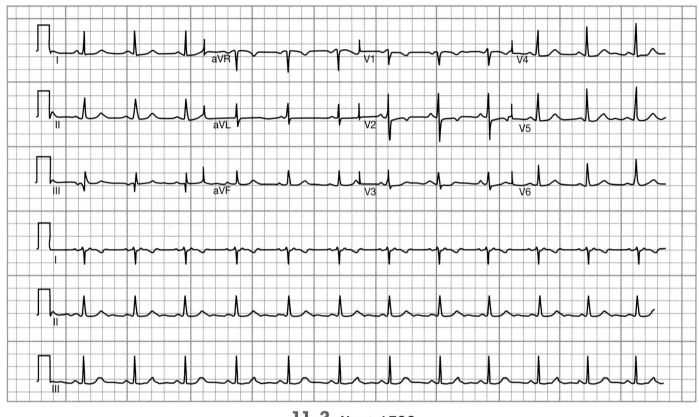

25mm/s	Med:			
10mm/mV		Wt: 156 lbs. Ht:		
100Hz	Sex: M	Race: Cauc		
Pgn	Loc: 12	Room:		
v206	Option: 14			
	Vent. rate	73	BMP	NORMAL SINUS RHYTHM
Cart:	PR interval	137	ms	NORMAL ECG
Tech:	QRS duration	80	ms	
Order number:	QT/QTc =	388/426	ms	
Secondary ID:	P–R–T axes	28–34–58	58	

11-3 Normal ECG

Courtesy of Edward Vandenberg, University of Nebraska Medical Center

An echocardiogram confirms that he has concentric left ventricular hypertrophy and a ventricular ejection value < 60%. The echocardiogram from Mr. Jones can be seen on the right.

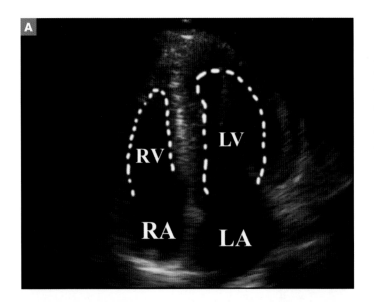

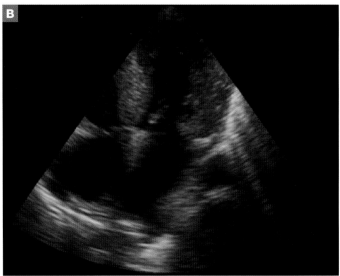

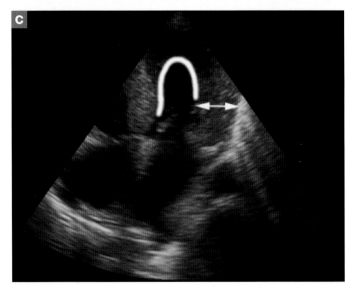

11-4 Echocardiograms of (A) normal heart, and (B and C) thickened left ventricle wall

Courtesy of Geoffrey Hayden, Medical University of South Carolina

Mr. Jones is given furosemide (Lasix), a diuretic medication that reduces water and sodium reabsorption from the loop of Henle. It is used for patients with left-sided heart failure.

When asked how he feels right now, he says, "Thanks—I feel okay, but I can't go. I tried this urinal thing, but nothing is coming out. And now I have a pain in my lower stomach."

The nurse catheterizes Mr. Jones with a Foley catheter, and urine begins to flow into the catheter bag. "Usually I have to go all the time," says Mr. Jones, "but then when I do go—it starts and then it stops and I just cannot empty my bladder! I hate this tube thing, but it sure relieves the pain in my bladder!" Later that day Mr. Jones is given a digital rectal exam and a prostate-specific antigen (PSA) blood test. He learns that he has benign prostatic hypertrophy (BPH).

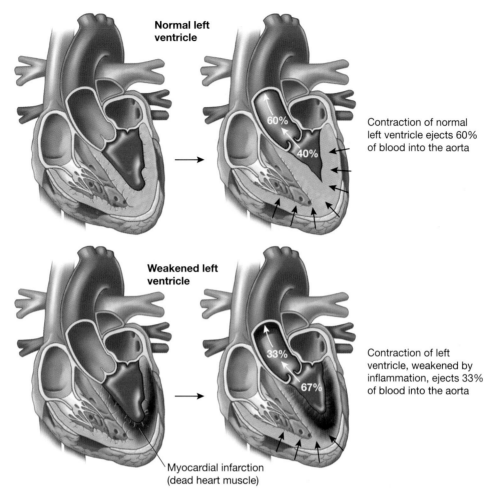

Normal left ventricle

60%

40%

Contraction of normal left ventricle ejects 60% of blood into the aorta

Weakened left ventricle

33%

67%

Contraction of left ventricle, weakened by inflammation, ejects 33% of blood into the aorta

Myocardial infarction (dead heart muscle)

11-5 Comparison of normal and weakened left ventricle wall

References

- American Urological Association. "BPH Guidelines."
  http://www.auanet.org/content/guidelines-and-quality-care/clinical-guidelines.cfm?sub=bph.

- Family Practice Notebook. "Left Ventricular Hypertrophy Related EKG Changes."
  http://www.fpnotebook.com/cv/Myocardium/LftVntrclrHyprtrphyRltdEkgChngs.htm.

- Global Initiative for Chronic Obstructive Lung Disease. http://www.goldcopd.com.

- Global Medical Education Project. "Left Ventricular Hypertrophy."
  http://lifeinthefastlane.com/ecg-library/basics/left-ventricular-hypertrophy.

- Heart Failure Online. http://www.heartfailure.org.

- Heart Failure Society of America. "Heart Failure Treatment Guidelines." http://www.heartfailureguideline.org.

Questions

1 What is COPD? What are the symptoms? What causes it?

2 How are chronic bronchitis and emphysema related to COPD?

3 An agonist drug binds to the drug receptor and mimics the actions of an endogenous substance (naturally occurring in the body). Where are the β_2 receptors in the body, and what is the endogenous substance that binds to them? What happens as a result? Explain the difference between selective and nonselective beta blockers.

4 Anticholinergic drugs bind to cholinergic receptors. Acetylcholine is the endogenous substance that binds to cholinergic receptors. But inflammatory mediators (histamine, bradykinin, eicosanoids) also stimulate cholinergic receptors. What happens when cholinergic receptors are stimulated in the airways? Why would oral anticholinergic drugs such as the over-the-counter antihistamine diphenhydramine (Benadryl) be dangerous for a patient with COPD but the inhaled anticholinergic drug Atrovent (ipratropium) be beneficial?

5 What do the arterial blood gas values suggest?

6 What causes left-sided heart failure? What symptoms of heart failure does Mr. Jones have?

7 Lasix is a diuretic medication that reduces water reabsorption from the loop of Henle. It is used with patients who have left-sided heart failure. Why would a diuretic affecting the loop of Henle help Mr. Jones?

8 How does a Foley catheter work?

9 What are the symptoms of BPH, and what causes it?

10 What did Mr. Jones do to cause his current symptoms?

The Ice Fishing Derby

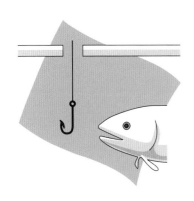

It was the day of the Crystal Lake Ice Fishing Derby. Pierre Larouc had been on the ice for six hours. He had just finished the traditional derby lunch of hot coffee, baked beans, hot dogs, and s'mores cooked over a fire on the ice. After he had two beers and sat in his ice fishing shanty with a cigar to relax, flags went up simultaneously on three lines. As he ran to check his catch, he felt a crushing pain just below his sternum and radiating to the left shoulder and jaw.

He put his hand on his chest inside his clothes and noticed something was missing. Pierre took a small canister from his pocket and sprayed it into his mouth. Just as fast as the pain came on, it stopped, and he pulled up three of the largest pike he had ever caught in February. When he got home to show his catch to his wife, Suzy, he found a note from a neighbor stating that she had taken Suzy to the emergency room because she was dizzy and "lightheaded."

References

- Alaeddini, J. 2012. "Angina Pectoris." *eMedicine* (February 14). http://emedicine.medscape.com/article/150215-overview.

1 What did Pierre spray into his mouth? What did it do for his cardiac muscle?

2 What pathophysiological problem does Pierre have? What causes it?

3 Did Pierre have a myocardial infarction (MI, or heart attack)? What leads you to this conclusion?

4 What were the triggers of the pain that Pierre experienced? Explain the mechanism of each.

5 When Suzy was seen in the ER, her blood pressure was 90/58. Her normal blood pressure is 115/70. What do you think caused this episode of hypotension?

_____

_____

_____

_____

_____

_____

_____

6 What precautions must Pierre remember to take in the future?

_____

_____

_____

_____

_____

_____

_____

_____

_____

_____

_____

_____

CASE
13

"My Professor Makes No Sense!"

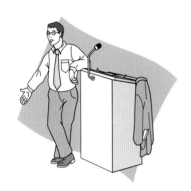

Sophomore Susan Jones is in the Student Advisory Center meeting with her tutor. "I don't know what else to do. I go to every class. I read the book. I take careful notes. I even tried taping the class like you suggested. I still got a D on the exam last week. My professor makes no sense! Everyone says so. Here—listen to the tape."

The tutor clicks on the tape, thinking that this would be a teachable moment to help Susan with active listening and note-taking skills. The professor starts: "Inflammatory mediators released immediately from mast cells include histamine, neutrophil chemotactic factor, and eosinophil chemotactic factor of anaphylaxis (known as ECF-A)."

"Well this is difficult material," says the tutor.

"I know," says Susan, "but go on with the tape!"

The professor on the tape continues "And sero, seri, Suzie...uh...platelets...uh so the cells go and do it... uh, okay, class, you can go now."

"This was right before the last exam!" says Susan. We're lost, and we have another exam in three weeks. Does he have Alzheimer's or something? He should retire!"

With concern, the tutor makes a call to the professor's department and finds out that the professor had been hospitalized earlier that day.

Meanwhile, the professor is having tests at the hospital emergency department. Following is what is known about the professor:

He reports that he has been having episodes for the past two months in which he forgets what he is about to say during a lecture and cannot find the words. His vision dims. Episodes typically last about two minutes. He thought he was having either anxiety or orthostatic hypotension from his Zestril (lisinopril), prescribed for hypertension, so he stopped taking it. Today, his episode lasted almost 10 minutes. He has not been taking his Lipitor (atorvastatin), prescribed for high cholesterol, over the past month because he says, "I've been following my diabetic diet" for pre–type 2 diabetes mellitus, diagnosed six months ago. He takes Inderal (propranolol, purchased over the Internet) every morning before class to reduce his anxiety while speaking.

- Smoker: 1 pack/day

- Height: 5'11"

- Weight: 195 lbs.

The Professor's Lab Values

Test	Value	SI Units	Reference Values	SI Units
Glucose (4 hrs post-prandial)	165 mg/dL	9.16 mmol/L	< 140 mg/dL	< 7.8 mmol/L
HbA1c	10.4%		< 6%	
LDL cholesterol	175 mg/dL	4.5 mmol/L	60–130 mg/dL (ideal is < 100 mg/dL)	1.5–3.4 mmol/L (ideal is < 2.6 mmol/L)
Blood pressure	156/94 mmHg		120/80 mmHg	40–55 g/L
Resting pulse	52 bpm		60–90 (lower in athletes)	

Below is a Doppler ultrasound image of the professor's left (normal) carotid artery. The image is obtained from the reflection or transmission of ultrasonic waves through the carotid artery.

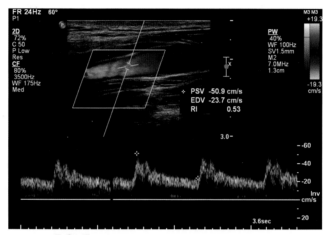

13-1 Doppler of left carotid artery

Courtesy of Mustapha Azzam, MD, 2008

Below is a Doppler ultrasound image of the professor's right carotid artery.

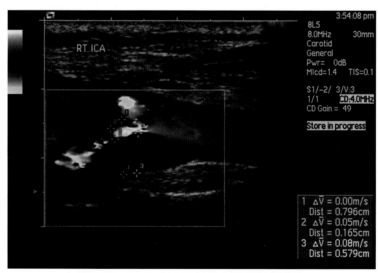

13-2 Doppler of right carotid artery

S.K. Kakkos and G. Geroulakous, *PLOS Medicine* 2, no. 4, e79doi:10.1371/journal.pmed.0020079

Below, left, is an angiogram image of the professor's left (normal) carotid artery. On the right is an angiogram image of the professor's right carotid artery. A catheter was inserted into his femoral artery and moved to the carotid artery. A radio opaque contrast material then was injected. The contrast material blocks the passage of X-rays and allows the visualization of carotid arteries on a fluoroscope (an X-ray machine that projects images on a television monitor).

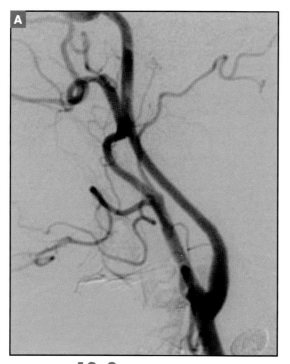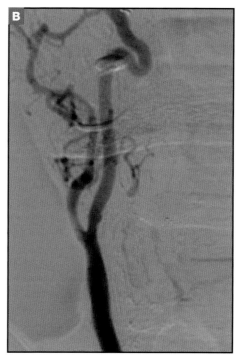

13-3 **Carotid artery**   (A) Left, normal; (B) Right, narrowed by plaque

Courtesy of Intermountain Medical Imaging, Boise, ID

References

- Johnston, S. C., R. M. Rothwell, M. N. Nguyen-Huynh, M. F. Giles, J. S. Elkins, A. L. Bernstein, and S. Sidney. 2007. "Validation and Refinement of Scores to Predict Very Early Stroke Risk after Transient Ischaemic Attack." *Lancet* 369: 283–292.

- MDCalc.com. "ABCD2 Score for Transient Ischemic Attack (TIA)." http://www.mdcalc.com/abcd2-score-for-tia.

- Medline Plus. "Transient Ischemic Attack." http://www.nlm.nih.gov/medlineplus/transientischemicattack.html.

- National Institute of Neurological Disorders and Stroke. "Transient Ischemic Attack." http://www.ninds.nih.gov/disorders/tia/tia.htm.

- Smale, Laurie. "Panic Free/Fearless Public Speaking." http://www.panicfreepublicspeaking.com.au/freetips.html.

1   a. What problem caused the professor's symptoms?

    b. What are his risk factors for this problem?

    c. What other symptoms are characteristic of this problem?

2   How do the symptoms of this problem vary by the area of the brain affected?

3   What do the glucose and HbA1c values suggest related to control of the professor's diabetes?

4   What signs are revealed by the tape recording, and what do they indicate? How high is the professor's risk
    for a cerebral vascular accident (CVA, or stroke)? See **http://www.mdcalc.com/abcd2-score-for-tia** for help.

5 How will the professor's problems be treated?

6 Why does the professor have a slow pulse of 52?

Joey Makes the Travel Soccer Team

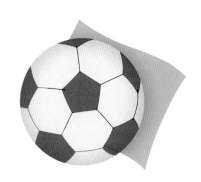

Joey Santos, age 9, made the Roadrunners travel soccer team and was excited to be able to play right wing. At 5'3" (160 cm) and 105 lbs. (48 kg), he was taller and thinner than most of his teammates aged 9–11. Practices began August 15, and his first away game was against the Saguaros at Marana. Joey had lost weight in the past month, and he always seemed to be hungry and thirsty. He had an appointment with the eye doctor in the next week because he told his mother that sometimes the blackboard in the classroom was blurry. Last week he had a cold, followed by a "stomach bug." He seemed to be better, and now he said he just had "butterflies." "Just nerves," thought his mother. She was worried about him getting dehydrated in the late summer Arizona air, so she packed coconut water for him. "This is new, Joey," she said. "It tastes great, and it has potassium, which is really good for you."

Joey played well during the first quarter, defending five shots on goal and getting a goal himself. He was hot, and he was sweaty. He drank a bottle of coconut water and went out for the second quarter. He felt tired and a little queasy, and his stomach began to hurt. Joey started coughing and staggering. His coach noticed something was wrong, so he brought him to the bench. A teammate mentioned that Joey's breath smelled a little funny. "Have some more water, Joey" the coach said. After slowly sipping a second bottle of coconut water, Joey stood up, clutched his stomach and passed out. "He's breathing funny!" shouted his coach. He called 911. Joey's pulse was hard to feel, so the coach put his head on Joey's chest and could tell Joey's heart was beating very fast. The paramedics arrived in four minutes. They used a glucometer to measure his blood glucose level, which was 361 mg/dL (20 mmol/L). They immediately gave him 10 units of insulin IV bolus and transported him to the emergency department.

References

- University of California, San Francisco, Diabetes Teaching Center. "Diabetes Education Online." http://dtc.ucsf.edu.

- Wofsdorf, J., N. Glaser, and M. A. Sperling. 2006. "Diabetic Ketoacidosis in Infants, Children, and Adolescents: A Consensus Statement from the American Diabetes Association." *Diabetes Care* 29, no. 5: 1150–1159. http://care.diabetesjournals.org/content/29/5/1150.full.

- Young, G.M. 2012. "Pediatric Diabetic Ketoacidosis." *eMedicine* (March 9). http://emedicine.medscape.com/article/801117-overview.

1 What disease did Joey likely develop over the past month? What leads you to this conclusion?

2 Describe the pathophysiology of Joey's disease, and explain how it differs from other forms of the disease.

3 What are the early symptoms of this disease in children?

4 What is the etiology of this disease in children? Discuss genetic and environmental factors that play a role in development of the disease.

5 What complication of this disease does Joey have *now*? What is the pathophysiology of this complication and possible consequences (sequelae)?

6   What are four goals in treating Joey for this complication? How will Joey be treated? Explain how his treatment will affect the pathophysiology of his disease.

_____

_____

_____

_____

_____

_____

_____

7   What is the composition of coconut water? What electrolyte imbalance could Joey have experienced because he consumed coconut water for rehydration?

_____

_____

8   When Joey arrived at the emergency department, he was assessed for cerebral edema. What is cerebral edema, and why was he at risk for it? How would he be treated to reduce this risk?

_____

_____

_____

_____

_____

_____

_____

_____

_____

_____

_____

9 Use the following template to make a concept map illustrating the relationships among the triggers, symptoms, and pathophysiology of Joey's problem.

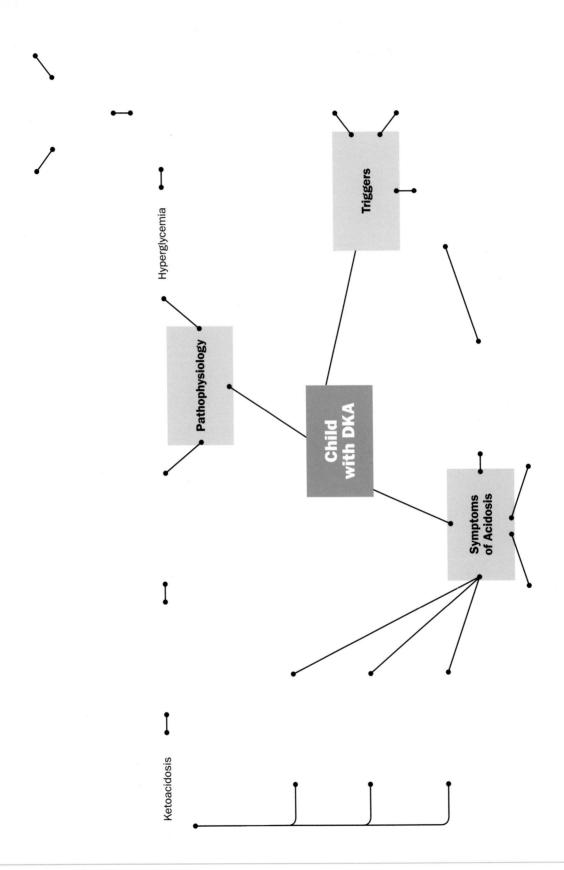

14-1 Concept map of relationships

Unmade Beds
at the B&B

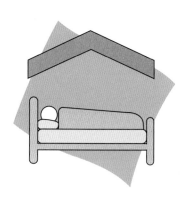

Jane and John (fraternal twins, age 56) and their spouses bought a bed-and-breakfast (B&B) a year ago. The year was stressful while they secured business loans, renovated the 150-year-old farmstead, and developed a business and marketing plan. Next month will be the grand opening of the 16-room B&B. Today the couples are reviewing the year and anticipating the future.

Jane says, "I'm exhausted—as I have been for the past month. I know my job is to get the beds ready, but I'm so fatigued it takes me half an hour to get each bed changed. That's quite a workout. I get out of breath! Now my back is bothering me, and I have an appointment in an hour for an MRI at the hospital."

At this, John interrupts and says, "I'm coming with you. I have this sharp pain running from my left shoulder up my neck and down my arm. I think I'll get checked out at the emergency room. All this painting is taking its toll."

John and Jane both have ECGs and blood tests and get MRIs.

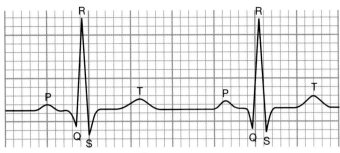

15-1 John's ECG

Courtesy of www.anaesthetist.com

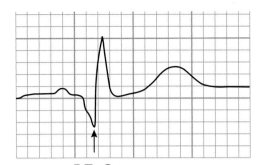

15-2 Jane's ECG

Courtesy of www.anaesthetist.com

John's Selected Lab Values				
	Value	**SI Units**	**Reference Range**	**SI Units**
Creatine phosphokinase (CK)	98 units/L		55–170 units/L	
CK-MB/CK isoenzyme	0%		0% of total CK	
Myoglobin	27 ng/ml	1.54 mmol/L	< 90 ng/ml	< 5.14 nmol/L
Troponin T	Not detected		< 0.2 ng/ml	< 0.2 mcg/L

Jane's Selected Lab Values				
	Value	**SI Units**	**Reference Range**	**SI Units**
Creatine phosphokinase (CK)	148 units/L		30–135 units/L	
CK-MB/CK isoenzyme	4%		0% of total CK	
Myoglobin	30 ng/ml	1.7 nmol/L	< 65 ng/ml	< 3.71 nmol/L
Troponin T	3.2 ng/ml	3.2 mcg/L	< 0.2 ng/ml	< 0.2 mcg/L

An MRI (magnetic resonance image) is a diagnostic imaging technique whereby the patient is put in a strong, uniform magnetic field. Protons absorb energy from the magnetic field and then emit radio waves as their excitation decays. These radiofrequency signals are converted into three-dimensional images. MRIs do not expose patients to ionizing radiation.

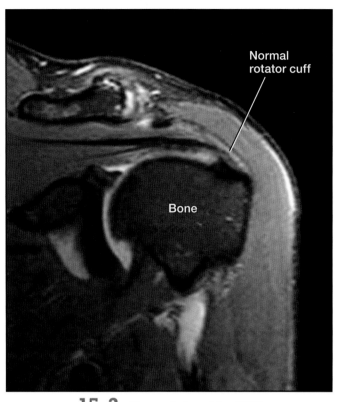

15-3 **Normal shoulder MRI**

Courtesy of Intermountain Medical Imaging, Boise, Idaho

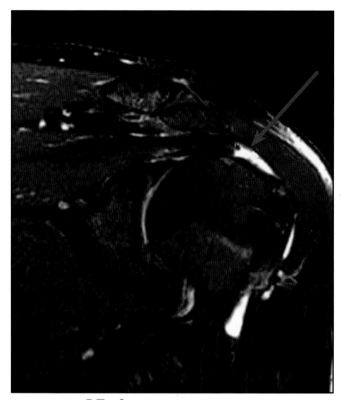

15-4 **John's shoulder MRI**

Courtesy of Intermountain Medical Imaging, Boise, Idaho

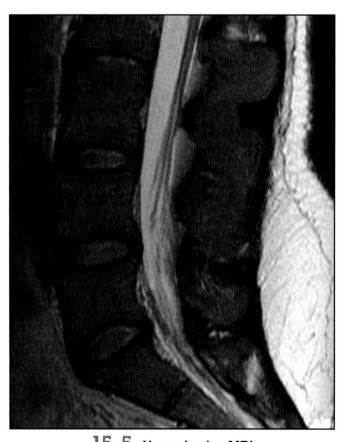

15-5 **Normal spine MRI**

Courtesy of Intermountain Medical Imaging, Boise, Idaho

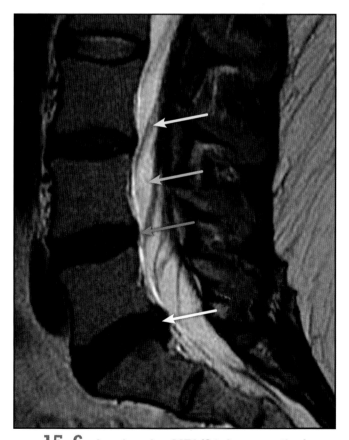

15-6 **Jane's spine MRI (S1 degeneration)**

Courtesy of Intermountain Medical Imaging, Boise, Idaho

References

- American Heart Association. http://www.heart.org/HEARTORG.

- Go Red for Women. http://www.goredforwomen.org.

- National Heart, Lung, and Blood Institute. "What Is a Coronary Calcium Scan?" http://www.nhlbi.nih.gov/health/dci/Diseases/cscan/cscan_whatis.html.

1 What problem can these selected lab values detect? What is the significance of each lab value? How could these lab values change over time?

_____

_____

_____

_____

_____

_____

_____

_____

2 What do John's ECG and lab values suggest? Are they normal or abnormal?

_____

_____

_____

3 What do Jane's ECG and lab values suggest? Are they normal or abnormal?

_____

_____

_____

4 To what could the red arrow on John's MRI be pointing?

_____

5 To what do the red, blue, yellow, and white arrows on Jane's MRI point?

_____

_____

6 What are gender-related differences in John's and Jane's symptoms?

_____

_____

_____

_____

_____

_____

7 What treatments/medications will John need?

_____

_____

8 What further assessments and treatments/medications will Jane need?

_____

_____

_____

_____

_____

_____

_____

_____

_____

_____

_____

A Failed Preschool Art Project

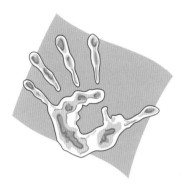

Justin Jones, age 4, is being seen in a pediatric hospital clinic. Mrs. Jones says, "Tuesday was Justin's first day of preschool. The children made handprint cards for their parents. Justin's teacher sent a note home to tell us that Justin's project didn't turn out too well because he doesn't have any fingerprints! We were bringing Justin to the clinic today anyway because he just doesn't seem to be growing. He is so much smaller than the other children in his class. And look at us—we're both tall! He has some kind of skin allergy on his arms, too. But now we're more worried about why he has no fingerprints!"

Justin appears small for his age. All other physical parameters appear within normal limits. His mother reports that Justin "has a good appetite, but he gets stomach pains and then diarrhea about two hours after he eats. The diarrhea is nasty. It's sort of frothy, and it floats!" He has patches of severe itchy skin on his upper arms, and his fingerprint ridges, though present, are faint.

Justin undergoes an endoscopic exam, and a biopsy is taken from his jejunum.

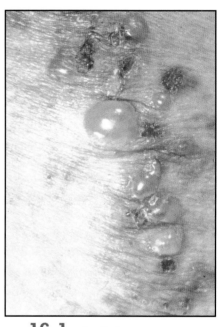

16-1 **Justin's upper arm**

Dermatology Nursing 16, no. 1 (2004): 31.
Reprinted with permission of the publisher,
Jannetti Publications, www.dermatologynursing.net.

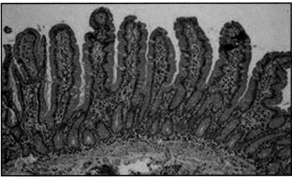

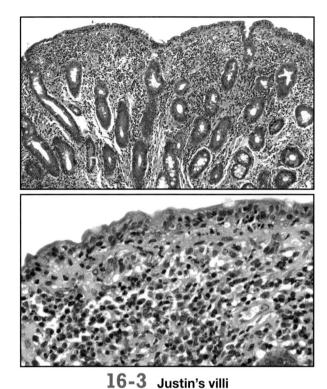

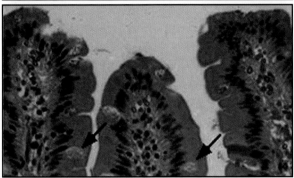

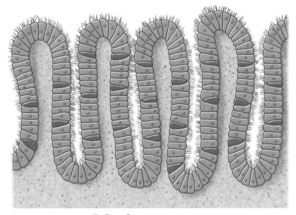

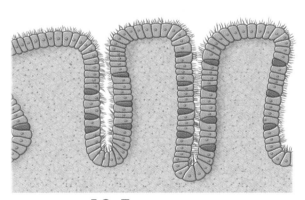

16-2 Normal villi

16-3 Justin's villi

16-4 Normal villi

16-5 Justin's villi

References

- American Celiac Disease Alliance. http://www.americanceliac.org.

- American Gastroenterological Association (AGA) Institute. "AGA Institute Medical Position Statement on the Diagnosis and Management of Celiac Disease." http://www.gastro.org/mobiletools/mobile-guidelines/aga-institute-medical-position-statement-on-the-diagnosis-and-management-of-celiac-disease.

- American Gastroenterological Association Patient Center. "Understanding Celiac Disease." http://www.gastro.org/patient-center/digestive-conditions/celiac-disease.

- Celiac Disease Foundation. http://www.celiac.org.

- Fasano, A. 2009. "Surprises from Celiac Disease." *Scientific American* 301: 54–61. http://www.nature.com/scientificamerican/journal/v301/n2/box/scientificamerican0809-54_BX3.html.

1 a. In what percentile for height and weight is Justin? _____

   b. Plot Justin's growth on the chart below. Enter "Justin Jones" after name. Enter record # as 3120.
   Enter the following data for:

Date	Age	Weight	Stature
8/1/11	2 yr 2 mo	12 kg	86 cm
9/1/12	3 yr 3 mo	12 kg	90 cm
9/7/13	4 yr 3 mo	14 kg	99 cm

NAME _____

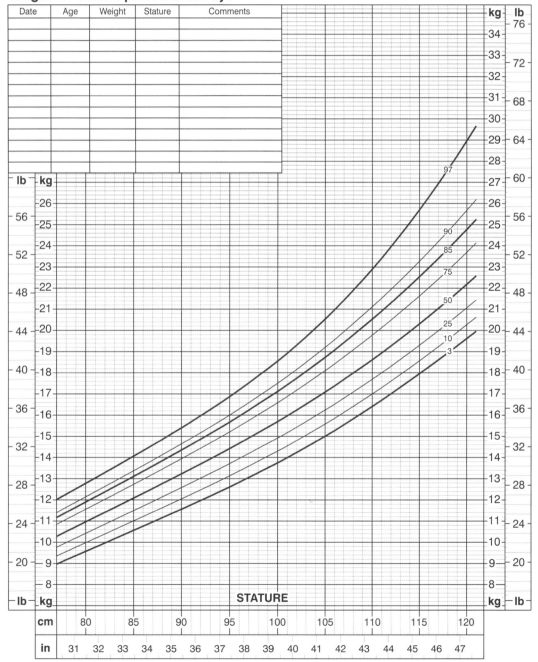

Weight-for-stature percentiles: Boys

RECORD # _____

Published May 30, 2000 (modified 10/16/00).
SOURCE: Developed by the National Center for Health Statistics in collaboration with
the National Center for Chronic Disease Prevention and Health Promotion (2000).
http://www.cdc.gov/growthcharts

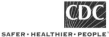

SAFER · HEALTHIER · PEOPLE™

2   Describe how Justin's villi differ from normal.

3   What functions of villi are impaired as a result of Justin's condition?

4   What caused the diarrhea? What is the technical term for this type of diarrhea?

5   How does Justin's skin differ from normal?

6   What condition does Justin have, and what causes it?

7 What is the etiology of this condition, and how frequent is it?

_____

_____

_____

8 What other disease is frequently associated with Justin's condition?

_____

_____

_____

_____

9 For which diseases will Justin be at increased risk over the long term?

_____

_____

_____

_____

_____

10 How can this condition be treated?

_____

_____

_____

_____

_____

_____

_____

The Reenactor

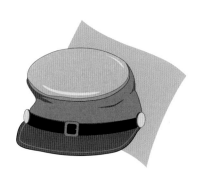

George Williams and his wife, Sharon, have been Civil War reenactors for more than 10 years. For the 150th anniversary of the Battle of Gettysburg, George got to play Daniel Sickles of the Union Army, and Sharon played a Gettysburg townswoman. More than 15,000 reenactors descended on the historic battlefield over the weekend before July 4th, and more than 50,000 spectators viewed the reenactments. The weather was as hot as during the actual battle July 2–6, 1863, with temperatures in the high 90s and high humidity.

Just like Sickles, George got impatient waiting for action and moved his Third Union Corps from Little Round Tops to the Peach Orchard. George commanded his corps to move, but then he slipped, fell, and gouged the right side of his calf on a rock. He was bleeding, hot, and tired. He sent Sharon a text, and she came up to Little Round Tops with an emergency kit. "Rather unlike the care the men actually got 150 years ago!" said George. "Well," said Sharon, "I've got to cut away those nice uniform pants I made you to see what you've done this time!" Sharon used the kit scissors and cut the wool fabric in four places to reveal the wound. "Ew!" said Sharon. "A 2-inch slash in your leg. Looks a bit dirty, too. What exactly did you cut it on?" George replied, "I slipped, and my leg just went into the rock." Sharon took off her apron and covered the wound to stop the bleeding. "This is too close to reality for me, George!" she said. But I think I can pull the cut back together if I use some of these butterfly bandages." With three butterfly bandages, Sharon was able to pull the edges of the wound together. "I think mostly your pride was hurt on this field, George!" she laughed. George got up and went back to his corps, rather proud of the state of his now especially realistic looking uniform. Sharon went back to her spot at the top of Seminary Ridge. The reenactment continued for another six hours. By 6 p.m., George found Sharon enjoying the postbattle barbeque. He was too tired to eat, so Sharon suggested they get in the truck and go back home, which was only an hour away.

When George and Sharon got home, George said "I really don't feel so well. Maybe I have a touch of heatstroke?" "Your head is cool, George. Let me take your temperature." George's temperature was 94.8°F (34.9°C). You really are a cool cucumber, George. You must have done a good job of keeping hydrated out there. I don't think it's heatstroke. Maybe you are just wiped out. Still, I better take you to the emergency room anyway and have your leg checked out."

When George got to the emergency department, his wound was assessed and described as a 5 cm simple soft-tissue laceration (i.e., it avoided the ligaments, muscle, and tendons in his calf). His vital signs were as follows:

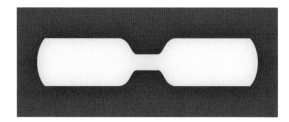

17-1 **Butterfly bandage**

- Temperature (oral): 94.8°F (34.9°C)
- Blood pressure: 110/68 (client's wife reports that his BP at home last week was 122/85)
- Heart rate: 90
- Respiratory rate: 24/min.
- Pulse oximetry (oxygen saturation): 98%

References

- Arlington National Cemetery Website. "Daniel Edgar Sickles." http://www.arlingtoncemetery.net/dsickles.htm.
- Capellan, O., and J. Hollander. 2003. "Management of Lacerations in the Emergency Department." *Emergency Medicine Clinics of North America* 21, no. 1 (February). https://secure.muhealth.org/~ed/students/articles/emcna_21_p205.pdf.
- Gabriel, A. 2011. "Wound Irrigation." *eMedicine* (May 19). http://emedicine.medscape.com/article/1895071-overview.
- Martin, G. S., D. M. Mannino, and S. Eaton, et al. 2003. "The Epidemiology of Sepsis in the United States from 1979 through 2000." *New England Journal of Medicine* 348, no. 16: 1546–1554.
- Rivers, Emanuel P., and Tom Ahrens. 2008. "Improving Outcomes for Severe Sepsis Shock: Tool for Early Identification of At-Risk Patients and Treatment Protocol." *Critical Care Clinics* 24, no. 3, Supplement 1 (July): 1–47. http://www.criticalcare.theclinics.com/issues?issue_key=S0749-0704(08)X0004-1.
- SEPSIS Know from Day 1. "What Is Procalcitonin?" http://www.sepsisknowfromday1.com/what-is-procalcitonin.php.
- Singhal, H. 2012. "Wound Infection Treatment and Management." *eMedicine* (January 6). http://emedicine.medscape.com/article/188988-treatment.
- Wedmore, I. S. 2005. "Wound Care: Modern Evidence in the Treatment of Man's Age-Old injuries." *EB Medicine*. http://www.ebmedicine.net/topics.php?paction=showTopic&topic_id=39.
- Zehtabchi, S. 2007. "Evidence-based Emergency Medicine/Critically Appraised Topic: The Role of Antibiotic Prophylaxis for Prevention of Infection in Patients with Simple Hand Lacerations." *Annals of Emergency Medicine* 49, no. 5: 682–289.e1.
- Zinn, S. P. "Medical Student LC: Module 1—Wound Care and Healing." http://www.medstudentlc.com/page.php?id=67.

Questions

1 How should individuals be taught to care for a laceration acquired "in the field," assuming medical care can be accessed within four to six hours?

_____

_____

_____

_____

_____

_____

_____

_____

_____

2 Describe the wound care George should receive upon reaching the emergency department.

_____

_____

_____

_____

_____

_____

_____

_____

_____

_____

_____

3 What is sepsis, and what are the early signs of sepsis from a laceration acquired in the field?

4 Was closing George's laceration in the field with butterfly bandages a good idea? Why or why not?

5 Using the diagrams on the next page as a guide, fill in the blanks to describe the three phases of wound healing and the role of the cellular "actors" involved.

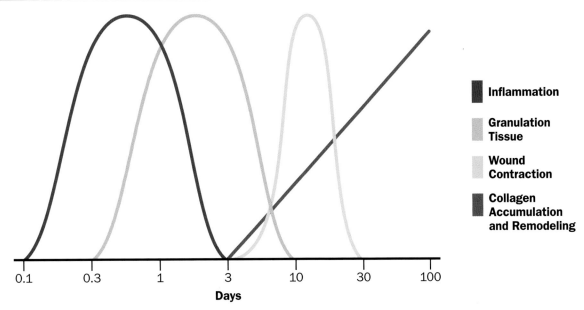

17-1 **Phases of wound healing**

Inflammation

Granulation
Tissue

Wound
Contraction

Collagen
Accumulation
and Remodeling

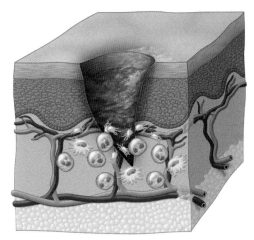 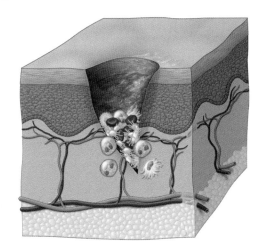

17-2 Phase 1: Inflammation; vascular and cellular processes

Platelets: _____

Injured blood vessels: _____

Venules: _____

Neutrophils (PMNs): _____

Macrophages: _____

Blood clot: _____

Exudate: _____

End result: _____

How long it lasts: _____

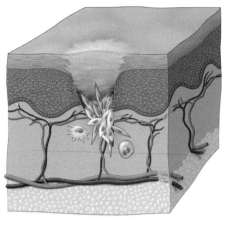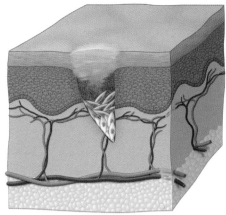

17-3 Phase 2: Proliferation and synthesis of new tissue

Macrophages: _____

Débridement: _____

Fibroblasts: _____

Granulation tissue: _____

Myofibroblasts: _____

End result: _____

How long it lasts: _____

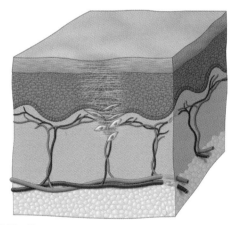

17-4 Phase 3: Remodeling and maturation

Fibroblasts: _____

Collagen: _____

Scar: _____

How long it lasts: _____

Name _____ Section _____

6 George has a soft-tissue laceration (i.e., it avoided the ligaments, muscle, and tendons in his calf) treated in the emergency department so that it could heal by tertiary intention (delayed primary closure). This treatment is used for contaminated wounds and has been shown to reduce risk of infection. Fill in the chart below with characteristics for each type of wound healing. See **http://www.medstudentlc.com/page.php?id=67** for help.

Type of Healing	Primary Intention	Secondary Intention	Tertiary Intention (Delayed Primary Closure)
Description			
Best for this type of wound			
Initial wound treatment			
Method of approximating wound margins			
Epithelialization			
Remodeling			
Final appearance and scarring			

7 Sickles was a controversial character before, during, and after the U.S. Civil War. What role did Sickles play during the Battle of Gettysburg, and did he help or hurt the Union side?

_____

_____

_____

_____

_____

_____

_____

_____

Never Too Old
to Learn a Bad Habit

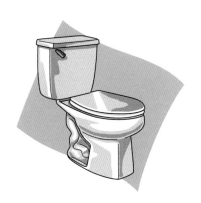

Olivia Gregor, age 98, decided on her own to enter the Evencare Assisted Living complex. Other than hypothyroidism (kept in control with thyroid replacement hormone for the past 50 years) her only health problems are open-angle glaucoma and macular degeneration. "Between the two, I really can't see much at all—especially the buttons on the phone and the microwave," she says, "but I'm lucky because I still have perfect memory, a good appetite (especially for dark chocolate!), and a sense of humor." Ms. Gregor settled in easily and formed a fast friendship with three sisters, "the Goodwin Girls," 20 years her junior.

Ms. Gregor uses prescription eyedrops (Xalatan) in her eyes every day to control her optic pressure. Her visual fields are tested frequently; she has lost a modest amount of peripheral vision, most of which happened before she was diagnosed at age 80. She also has lost a significant amount of central vision. She was "enjoying life" in Florida for five years and did not have her eyes examined during that time. She relies on her remaining peripheral vision to navigate her surroundings.

A month after arriving, Ms. Gregor developed a fever of 99°F and an itching and burning sensation when she urinated. Her urine developed an orange color and had a strong odor.

References

- Mayo Foundation for Research and Education. "Urinary Tract Infection." http://www.mayoclinic.com/health/urinary-tract-infection/DS00286.

- Shoff, W. H., and V. Batuman. 2012. "Asymptomatic Bacteriuria." *Medscape Reference.* http://emedicine.medscape.com/article/2059290-overview.

- Todar, K. 2012. "The Control of Microbial Growth." In *Todar's Online Textbook of Bacteriology.* Madison: University of Wisconsin, Department of Bacteriology. http://www.textbookofbacteriology.net/control.html.

1   What is open-angle glaucoma, and how does it affect vision?

_____

_____

_____

_____

2   What is macular degeneration, and how does it affect vision?

_____

_____

_____

_____

_____

_____

3   What is the most likely cause of Olivia Gregor's new problem—fever with itching and burning during urination?

_____

_____

_____

_____

_____

4   How can this new problem be treated?

_____

_____

_____

_____

5 Ms. Gregor's new problem resolves with treatment. But three weeks later her symptoms return. What is the likely cause of the return of her symptoms?

6 Olivia Gregor is treated again and responds rapidly. Over the course of the next six months, her symptoms return three more times. Each time the same antibiotic leads to prompt resolution of her symptoms. What do you think is going on?

7 Ms. Gregor has now been healthy for the past four months. However, her last urine culture was positive for bacteria—but she has no symptoms whatsoever. What treatment does she need?

"My Heart Is in My Stomach!"

CASE 19

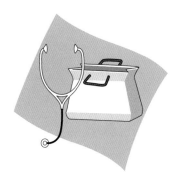

Mrs. V., age 52, comes into the hospital walk-in clinic and says, "My 6-year-old granddaughter got a medic kit for her birthday. She was using the stethoscope to hear my heartbeat, and she couldn't find it—it *is* a toy after all. But then she put the stethoscope on my stomach and said she heard a loud heartbeat. I can feel it too, just above my navel. Is it possible that my heart is in the wrong place? My granddaughter is telling everyone, 'Grandma has a baby in her tummy just like mommy! You can feel the heartbeat!'"

The notes from the triage nurse indicate the following:

- Female, age 52
- BP: 176/94 mm Hg
- Height (self-reported): 5'2" (157.5 cm)
- Weight (self-reported): 165 lbs. (74.8 kg)
- Smoker: one to two packs per day for 33 years

- Heart rate: 88 with occasional PVCs (one per minute)
- History of high cholesterol
- Last period was three months ago
- Pulsing mass above umbilicus, upper left of midline, palpable when supine.

A physician's assistant (PA) sees Mrs. V., takes a pregnancy test, and then orders an X-ray.

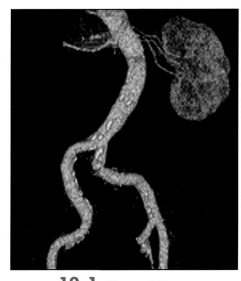

19-1 Normal X-ray
Courtesy of www.pennhealth.com

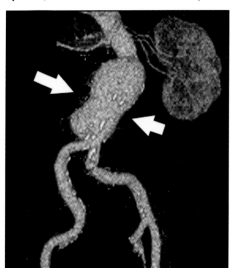

19-2 Mrs. V.'s X-ray
Courtesy of www.pennhealth.com

A multirow CT angiogram scan is then ordered for Mrs. V. This type of CT scan has multiple rows of detectors. Through a process called volume rendering, the final image appears three-dimensional.

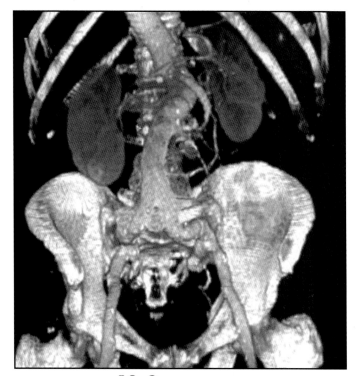

19-3 **Normal scan**

Courtesy of Madison Radiologists, http://www.madisonradiologists.com

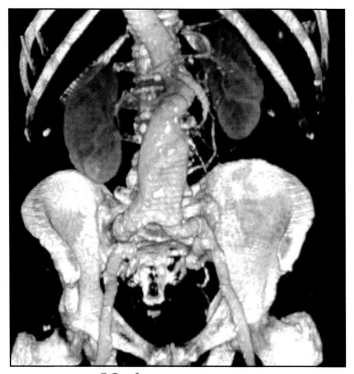

19-4 **Mrs. V.'s CT scan**

Courtesy of Madison Radiologists, http://www.madisonradiologists.com

References

- Pearce, W. H. 2011. "Abdominal Aortic Aneurysm." *eMedicine* (October 31). http://emedicine.medscape.com/article/1979501-overview.

- University of Pennsylvania Health System, Department of Radiology. "Abdominal Aortic Aneurysm." *PennMedicine*. http://www.uphs.upenn.edu/radiology/patient/services/ir/info/aaa.html.

- U.S. Department of Health and Human Services, Agency for Healthcare Research and Quality (AHRQ). "Screening: Abdominal Aortic Aneurysm." http://www.ahrq.gov/clinic/uspstf/uspsaneu.htm.

1   Why was a pregnancy test ordered for Mrs. V.?

2   What does Mrs. V.'s X-ray show? (*Hint*: X-rays show calcification. To what do the arrows point?)

3   What does Mrs. V.'s CT scan show?

4   What does Mrs. V. have? What risk factors and symptoms are associated with this condition in men and in women?

5 If Mrs. V. does nothing about this, what might happen to her?

_____

_____

_____

_____

_____

_____

_____

_____

_____

_____

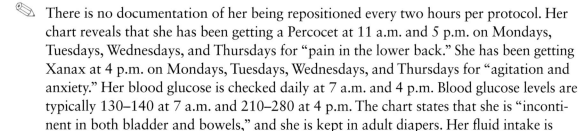

Stargazed

CASE 20

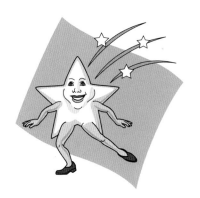

Mrs. Deland, age 78, has been living at Stargaze Health-Care Center for two months following hospitalization for a broken hip. She is frail and confined to bed and a wheelchair. She is moved to the wheelchair by use of a lift. Her medications include insulin for type 2 diabetes, lactulose for constipation, Percocet for pain as needed (contains acetaminophen as in Tylenol and oxycodone, an opioid), and Xanax as needed for anxiety. Nursing student John Smart has been observing the care of Mrs. Deland and has found the following, which he writes in his clinical course journal:

There is no documentation of her being repositioned every two hours per protocol. Her chart reveals that she has been getting a Percocet at 11 a.m. and 5 p.m. on Mondays, Tuesdays, Wednesdays, and Thursdays for "pain in the lower back." She has been getting Xanax at 4 p.m. on Mondays, Tuesdays, Wednesdays, and Thursdays for "agitation and anxiety." Her blood glucose is checked daily at 7 a.m. and 4 p.m. Blood glucose levels are typically 130–140 at 7 a.m. and 210–280 at 4 p.m. The chart states that she is "incontinent in both bladder and bowels," and she is kept in adult diapers. Her fluid intake is estimated at 2,000 cc/day.

A physical assessment on Monday reported that her skin had good turgor. Her pulse was 88 and strong. Her weight was 112 lbs. On Friday Mrs. Deland had poor skin turgor, a weak and thready pulse of 99, and her weight was 107 lbs. The water mug by her bedside is changed every four hours between 8 a.m. and 4 p.m. (three times a day, 24 oz. or 710 cc), and the amount remaining is measured. The record for Monday–Friday shows that no water was left in the water mug. Taken together with her fluid intake at meals, I estimate that Mrs. Deland is taking in more than 2,000 ccs of fluid per day. Her stools are reported to be formed and not watery.

John observes that during the week, Mrs. Deland has severe short-term memory problems but seems better on the weekends. For example, when the staff came in with the patient lift last Tuesday and Thursday during his clinical, Mrs. Deland could not remember what the lift was for, and "she was anxious as if she was seeing it for the first time." When he stopped in on Sunday to review her chart, he observed the staff placing Mrs. Deland in the lift, and she was calm and chatting. She spotted John and called out, "Hello, young man! Nice to see you again! They've come to take me to the toilet. Talk to you later!"

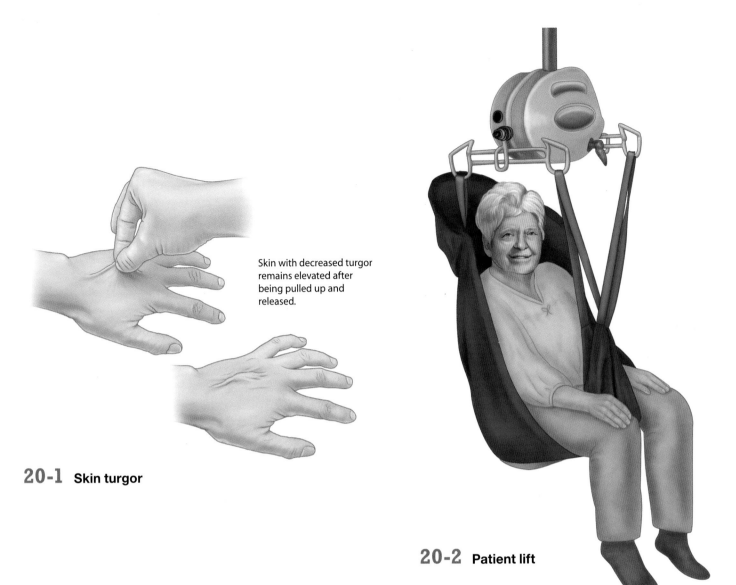

Skin with decreased turgor remains elevated after being pulled up and released.

20-1 Skin turgor

20-2 Patient lift

References

- Huang, L. H. 2012. "Dehydration." *eMedicine* (March 12). http://emedicine.medscape.com/article/906999-overview.

- Wixted, T. 2005. "A Theory about Why We Forget What We Once Knew." *Current Directions in Psychological Science* 14, no. 1: 6–9. http://wixtedlab.ucsd.edu/publications/wixted/Wixted_%282005%29.pdf.

Questions

1 Why do you think Mrs. Deland does *not* have short-term memory loss on the weekends? (*Hint:* Evaluate her medication schedule. Benzodiazepine sedatives, including Xanax, cause anterograde amnesia.)

_____

_____

_____

_____

2 Lactulose is a synthetic sugar that is not absorbed. It increases the osmolality of the stool. Osmolality is the concentration of osmotically active particles that attract water. The increased stool osmolality reduces water absorption from the colon, so more is left in the stool, thereby promoting laxation. What possible side effect do you think this could cause?

_____

_____

_____

3 Do you think Mrs. Deland is really incontinent? Why or why not? (*Hint*: Consider *when* the Percocet is given for "pain in the lower back.")

_____

_____

_____

_____

_____

4   What physical assessment results and lab values would you be interested in looking at?

_____

_____

_____

_____

_____

_____

_____

_____

_____

_____

_____

_____

_____

_____

_____

_____

_____

_____

5   A physical assessment of Mrs. Deland on Monday morning found that her skin had good turgor, and her pulse was 88 and strong. On Friday, however, Mrs. Deland had poor skin turgor and a weak and thready pulse of 99. A blood sample was taken on Friday at 4 p.m. Mrs. Deland was catheterized so a 24-hour urine sample could be analyzed. What do Mrs. Deland's blood and urine lab values suggest?

Name _____ Section _____

Mrs. Deland's Selected Lab Values

Test	Value	SI Units	Reference Range (nonfasting 4 p.m.)	SI Units
Glucose	240 mg/dL	13.3 mmol/L	< 200 mg/dL	< 11.1 mmol/L
BUN	18 mg/dL	6.4 mmol/L	7–18 mg/dL	2.5–6.4 mmol/L
Creatinine, serum	1.9 mg/dL	168 µmol/L	0.8–1.3 mg/dL	71–115 µmol/L
Bilirubin, total	1.2 mg/dL	20.5 µmol/L	0.1–1.0 mg/dL	1.71–17.1 µmol/L
Protein, total	7.5 g/dL	75 g/L	6.4–8.2 g/dL	64–82 g/L
Albumin	4.4 g/dL	44 g/L	3.4–5.0 g/dL	34–50 g/L
WBC	6.1 K/cmm		4.5–11.0 K/cmm	
RBC	5.5		4.00–5.20 K/cmm	
HGB	15.2 g/dL	152 g/L	12.0–16.0 g/dL	120–160 g/L
HCT	48.8%		36.0–46.0%	120–160 g/L
MCV	90 fL		80–100 fL	
MCH	31.2 pg		26.0–34.0 pg	
MCHC	33.7 g/dL	337 g/L	31.0–37.0 g/dL	310–370 g/L
Sodium	148 mEq/L	148 mmol/L	135–145 mEq/L	135–145 mmol/L
Potassium	4.9 mEq/L	4.9 mmol/L	3.5–5.1 mEq/L	3.5–5.1 mmol/L
Chloride	110 mEq/L	110 mmol/L	98–107 mEq/L	98–107 mmol/L
Calcium	10.0 mg/dL	2.5 mmol/L	8.5–10.5mg/dL	2.1–2.6 mmol/L

Mrs. Deland's Urine Test Results

Test	Value	SI Units	Reference Range (nonfasting 4 p.m.)	SI Units
Urine specific gravity	1.09		1.002–1.028	
Urine osmolality	1447 mOsm/kg	1447 mmol/kg	50–1,400 mOsm/kg	50–1,400 mmol/kg
Glucose	absent			
Microalbumin	absent			
Protein	absent			
Sodium	347 mEq/24h	347 mmol/L/24h	15–250 mEq/24 h	15–250 mmol/L/24h

6 Why didn't Mrs. Deland complain of thirst?

7 How will Mrs. Deland be treated?

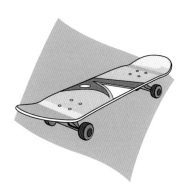

Daddy Learns to Do a 180

After a year of planning and three months of building work, the town skateboard park was ready to open. Gerome Lee, a computer programmer, and his son, Josh, a 16-year-old high school sophomore, were chairs of the skateboard park committee. Today they were the first to try it out. Josh easily navigated the vertical half-pipe ramp. "It's your turn, Dad!" he exclaimed.

Gerome, age 50, was quite the dude back in his day but hadn't actually been to a skateboard park before. "Show me how to do a 180 on the mini ramp first!" he asked his son.

"Like this, Dad!" Josh explained as he flipped around. Gerome did the same maneuver on the flats and then went for it. He did a perfect 180 on the mini ramp, then fell on his left hand. In severe pain, he dialed 911 on his cellphone.

When he arrived at the ER, Gerome was feeling much better. "I don't think anything is broken," he said. He was able to fill out a medical history record and reported the following:

- Chinese American male; height: 5'7" (170 cm); weight: 131 lbs. (59 kg)

- Smokes two packs of cigarettes daily

- Does not drink alcohol

- History of peptic ulcer at age 48; now self-medicating with OTC Prilosec for chronic gastric acid indigestion; took antacids daily for three years

- History of renal stones (two episodes in the past six months)

- History of childhood asthma; took oral prednisone between ages 8 and 12

- Lactose intolerant

- No other medications or supplements

- Exercise: occasional walks with dog

X-rays are taken of his left hand. There are no broken bones. There is, however, significant bone loss in the radial (lateral) aspect of the middle phalanx of both the index and middle fingers. He also has a brown spot on the middle phalanx on the index finger.

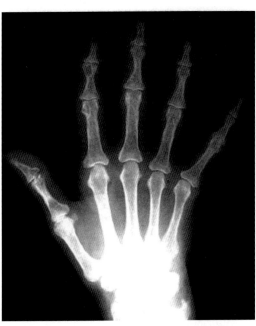

21-1 **X-ray of Gerome's right hand**

Courtesy www.radswiki.net

111

Below are his lab values.

Lab Test	Mr. Lee's Values	SI Units	Reference Values	SI Units
Calcium	11.2 mg/dL	2.8 mmol/L	8.5–10.5 mg/dL	2.1–2.6 mmol/L
Phosphorus	2.8 mg/dL	0.9 mmol/L	2.0–5.0 mg/dL	0.65–1.6 mmol/L
Potassium	5.3 mEq/L	5.3 mmol/L	3.2–5.2 mEq/L	3.2–5.2 mmol/L
Sodium	139 mEq/L	139 mmol/L	135–145 mEq/L	135–145 mmol/L
Alkaline phosphatase	145 U/Lm		25–125 U/L	
Alkaline phosphatase (bone fraction)	90 U/Lm		11–73 U/L	
Alkaline phosphatase (liver fraction)	50 U/Lm		0–93 U/L	
Thyroxine (T_4) total	10 ug/dL	128.7 nmol/L	4.6–10.5 µg/dL	59.2–135 nmol/L
TSH	2.5 uIU/L		0.4–4.2 µIU/L	
Parathyroid hormone (intact)	155 pg/mL	155 ng/L	10–65 pg/mL	10–65 ng/L

Gerome is sent for a Sestamibi scan of the neck. Sestamibi is a small protein radio-labeled with technetium-99 and injected into the vein. Technetium-99 is taken up by the parathyroid if there is a high concentration of parathyroid hormone, as in parathyroid tumors. The radioactivity can be detected and visualized by a gamma ray detecting scanner.

Following is an image from Gerome's scan.

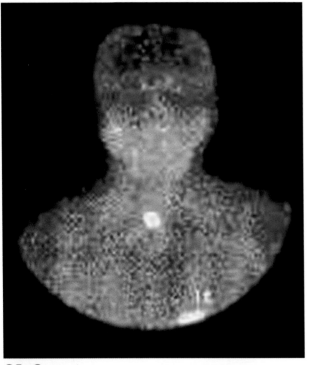

21-2 **Sestamibi scan of Gerome's neck**

Courtesy of J. Norman, MD, www.parathyroid.com

References

- Parathyroid.com. "Sestamibi Scans." http://www.parathyroid.com/sestamibi.htm.

- Salen, P. M. 2012. "Hyperparathyroidism." *Medscape Reference*. http://emedicine.medscape.com/article/766906-overview.

- WebMD. 2011. "Osteopenia." http://www.webmd.com/osteoporosis/tc/osteopenia-overview.

1 What is the difference between osteopenia and osteoporosis, and how can each be diagnosed?

2 What are the risk factors for bone loss in a 50-year-old man?

3 What do Gerome's lab values suggest? What symptoms support this conclusion?

_____

_____

_____

_____

_____

_____

_____

4 What does the Sestamibi scan of the neck region show?

_____

_____

_____

_____

_____

_____

_____

5 How will Gerome be treated?

_____

_____

_____

_____

_____

_____

_____

Neck Hygiene

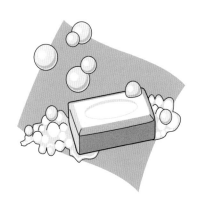

Charlene Woodstone is a 13-year-old girl in the eighth grade in a large junior high school in Texas. She is in the nurse's office in distress. "Ms. Jones told me to see you because I haven't got the dirt off my neck. I am *so* embarrassed! She talked to me in homeroom in front of everybody! I told her I *always* wash my neck, but she wouldn't even look at my neck up close or even *listen* to me!"

The information the school nurse has about Charlene is as follows:

- Age: 13
- Height: 5'3" (63 inches) (160 cm)
- Weight: 171 lbs. (77.5 kg)
- Age at menarche: 10
- Last period: "Three months ago? Periods not regular but frequent pelvic pain"
- Blood pressure: 138/82
- Pulse: 80

When asked if Charlene has any other concerns, she replies, "I dunno. I have hair where I shouldn't—like on the sides of my jaw and on my thumbs and toes. And my acne seems to be getting worse. I feel like a freak show." Charlene keeps her head down so her long hair covers the sides of her face. "The only thing I have going for me is singing soprano in the choir—but my choir teacher is on my case, too, because I sing with my head down."

The nurse notes that the "dirt" on Charlene's neck is actually an area of increased pigmentation (hyper-pigmentation) that has a thickened, rough surface (hyperkeratosis) that looks like velvet.

The nurse says, "Charlene, I'm going to call your mother and ask that she take you to a special doctor. I think you can be helped so the appearance of your skin improves and the hair on your face goes away."

Below is a photo of Charlene's face and neck:

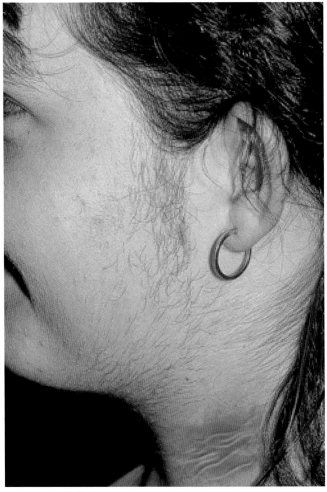

22-1 Charlene's face and neck

Journal of American Academy of Dermatology 55; reprinted in Gary M. White and Neil H. Cox,
Diseases of the Skin: A Color Atlas and Text, 2nd ed. Copyright Elsevier 2006.

References

- National Heart, Lungs, and Blood Institute. "Body Mass Index." http://www.nhlbisupport.com/bmi.

- National Heart, Lungs, and Blood Institute. "Metabolic Syndrome."
  http://www.nhlbi.nih.gov/health/health-topics/topics/ms.

- National Heart, Lungs, and Blood Institute. "Pocket Guide to Blood Pressure Measurement in Children."
  http://www.nhlbi.nih.gov/health/public/heart/hbp/bp_child_pocket/bp_child_pocket.pdf.

- University of Virginia Health System. "Polycystic Ovary Syndrome."
  http://uvahealth.com/services/diabetes-and-metabolism/conditions-treatments/11629.

- U.S. Department of Health and Human Services, Women's Office on Health. "Polycystic Ovary Syndrome (PCOS) Fact
  Sheet." http://www.womenshealth.gov/publications/our-publications/fact-sheet/polycystic-ovary-syndrome.cfm#f.

Questions

1 a. Assess Charlene's height and weight by calculating her body mass index (BMI) using the online calculator at **http://www.nhlbisupport.com/bmi**. Comment on your findings.

b. What are two risks associated with childhood obesity?

2 a. Assess Charlene's blood pressure reading. See **http://www.nhlbi.nih.gov/health/public/heart/hbp/bp_ child_pocket/bp_child_pocket.pdf** for help.

b. Can a diagnosis be made with a single blood pressure reading? If not, what are the guidelines?

3 a. What problem is causing the hyperpigmentation and hyperkeratosis on Charlene's neck? See **http://www.diabetesmonitor.com/b313.htm** and **http://www.dphhs.mt.gov/PHSD/Diabetes/pdf/Acan Brochure.pdf** for help.

b. What is the pathophysiology associated with the development of the hyperpigmentation?

4 What tests would diagnose the underlying causes of this problem? See **http://www.nhlbi.nih.gov/health/ health-topics/topics/ms** for help.

5 What problem is causing Charlene to have irregular periods, to experience pelvic pain, and to grow hair in unusual locations? See **http://www.diabetesmonitor.com/b219.htm** for help.

6 Charlene's new doctor orders blood tests and an ultrasound. Below are selected results. What do the results of Charlene's lab tests suggest? (*Hint:* Make a graph of her results and reference values.)

Fasting Blood Sample

	Charlene's Values	SI Units	Reference Range (non-fasting)	SI Units
Glucose	122 mg/dL	6.77 mmol/L	70–100 mg/dL	3.9–6.1 mmol/L
Triglycerides	275 mg/dL	3.11 mmol/L	15–150 mg/dL	0.17–1.7 mmol/L
LDL cholesterol	178 mg/dL	4.6 mmol/L	0.0–99.0 mg/dL	0.0–2.6 mmol/L
HDL cholesterol	35 mg/dL	0.9 mmol/L	> 40 mg/dL	> 1 mmol/L
C-reactive protein (CRP)	0.68 mg/dL	6.8 g/L	< 0.3 mg/dL	< 3 g/L

Glucose Tolerance Test

Time	Charlene's Values	SI Units	Reference Range (non-fasting)	SI Units
0 (fasting)				
Glucose	125 mg/dL	7 mmol/L	< 100 mg/dL	< 5.5 mmol/L
Insulin	7.7 µU/mL	54 pmol/L	< 10 µU/mL	< 69.5 pmol/L
1/2 hour				
Glucose	145 mg/dL	8 mmol/L	< 200 mg/dL	11.1 mmol/L
Insulin	78 µU/mL	542 pmol/L	40–70 µU/mL	278–486 pmol/L
1 hour				
Glucose	180 mg/dL	10 mmol/L	< 200 mg/dL	< 11.1 mmol/L
Insulin	99.9 µU/mL	694 pmol/L	50–90 µU/mL	347–625 pmol/L
2 hours				
Glucose	160 mg/dL	9 mmol/L	< 140 mg/dL	< 7.8 mmol/L
Insulin	98 µU/mL	680 pmol/L	6–50 µU/mL	35-347 pmol/L

Reference values from www.inciid.org

Below, left, is an ultrasound of Charlene's left ovary. The image was obtained from the reflection or transmission of ultrasonic waves through the ovary. The arrows point to numerous small cysts that fill the space. Below, right, is an ultrasound photo of a normal ovary with a mature follicle, midcycle.

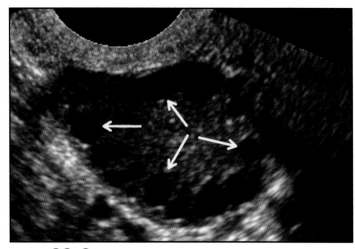

22-2 Ultrasound of Charlene's left ovary

Courtesy of William Herring, MD, www.learningradiology.com

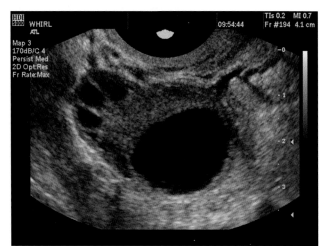

22-3 Ultrasound of normal ovary

D. Chizen and R. Pierson, Global Library of Women's Medicine *(ISSN: 1756-2228)* 2010; DOI 10.3843/GLOWM.10326
Reprinted with permission of Sapiens Publishing.

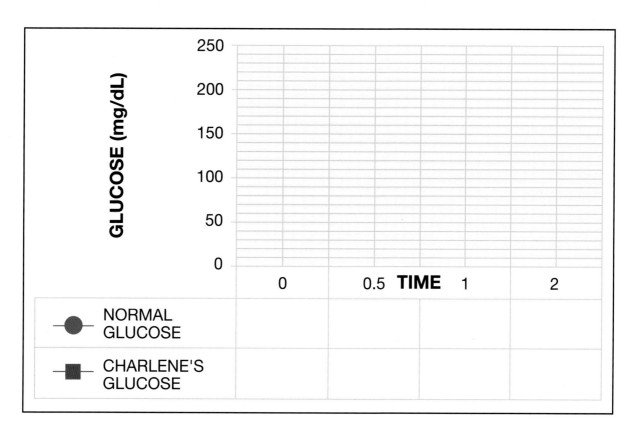

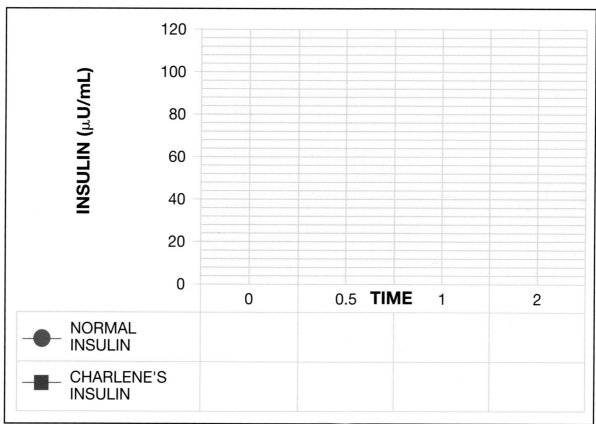

7 How will Charlene be treated?

The Trainer

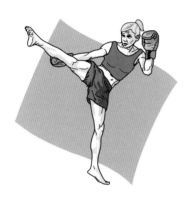

Margie O. is "50, fit, and fabulous." She celebrated her big 5-0 birthday by going to the health club and having a free, quick cholesterol check. Her trainer reported that her cholesterol was 222 mg/dL (5.7 mmol/L). "This is too high for someone as fit as you. I suggest you do double sets of your regimen for a month. Sign up for an extra kickboxing class. That will really burn calories and probably lower your cholesterol!" Margie tried this as well as eating a vegetarian low-fat diet. Although her weight hadn't changed, she thought her face was getting fatter—the first place she always gained.

The next month she asked her trainer to test her cholesterol again. "Wow—now it's up to 260, Margie! I think you should go to your doctor and have it tested."

Margie had a physical exam, mammogram, colonoscopy, and fasting blood test the following week. The results of her mammogram and colonoscopy were negative. Selected results of her fasting blood test are given on the next page.

Margie's Test Results

Test	Value	SI Units	Reference Range	SI Units
Glucose	78 mg/dL	4.3 mmol/L	70–100 mg/dL	3.9–6.1 mmol/L
BUN	8 mg/dL	2.8 mmol/L	7–18 mg/dL	2.5–6.4 mmol/L
Creatinine, serum	1.3 mg/dL	115 µmol/L	0.8–1.3 mg/dL	71–115 µmol/L
Bilirubin, total	1.0 mg/dL	17.1 µmol/L	0.1–1.0 mg/dL	1.71–17.1 µmol/L
Protein, total	7.5 g/dL	75 g/L	6.4–8.2 g/dL	64–82 g/L
Albumin	4.4 g/dL	44 g/L	3.4–5.0 g/dL	34–50 g/L
Alkaline phosphatase	123 U/L		50–136 U/L	
Aspartate amino-transferase/SGOT (AST/SGOT)	27 U/L		15–37 U/L	
Alanine amino-transferase/SGOT (ALT/SGOT)	40 U/L		30–65 U/L	
Gamma-glutamyl transferase (GGT)	39 U/L		1–94 U/L	
Cholesterol, total	260 mg/dL	6.7 mmol/L	50–199 mg/dL	1.3–5.2 mmol/L
Triglycerides	150 mg/dL	1.7 mmol/L	15–149 mg/dL	0.17–1.7 mmol/L
LDL (direct)	170 mg/dL	4.4 mml/L	0–99.0 mg/dL	0.0–2.6 mmol/L
HDL	60 gm/dL	1.6 mmol/L	> 40 mg/dL	> 1 mmol/L
WBC	7.1 K/cmm		4.5–11.0 K/cmm	
RBC	5.0 K/cmm		4.00–5.20 K/cmm	
Hemoglobin (HGB)	14.9 g/dL	149 g/L	12.0–16.0 g/dL	120–160 g/L
Hematocrit (HCT)	44.8 %		36.0–46.0%	2.1–2.6 mmol/L
Mean corpuscular volume (MCV)	90 fL		80–100 fL	
Mean corpuscular hemoglobin (MCH)	32.1 pg		26.0–34.0 pg	
Mean corpuscular hemoglobin concentration (MCHC)	31.2 g/dL	312 g/L	31.0–37.0 g/dL	310–370 g/L
Sodium	140 mEq/L	140 mmol/L	136–145 mEq/L	136–145 mmol/L
Potassium	4.6 mEq/L	4.6 mmol/L	3.5–5.1 mEq/L	3.5–5.1 mmol/L
Chloride	99 mEq/L	99 mmol/L	98–107 mEq/L	98–107 mmol/L
CO_2, total	26.9 mEq/L	26.9 mmol/L	21.0–32.0 mEq/L	21.0–32.0 mmol/L
T4, free	0.6 ng/dL	7.7 pmol/L	0.8–1.5 ng/dL	10.3–19.3 pmol/L
TSH	6.7 µIU/L		0.4-4.2 µIU/L	
Thyroid peroxidase antibody (TPO antibody)	1089		< 20 IU/mL	

References

- National Heart, Lung, and Blood Institute, National Cholesterol Education Program (NCEP). "Risk Assessment Tool for Estimating 10-Year Risk of Developing Hard CHD (Myocardial Infarction and Coronary Death)." http://hp2010.nhlbihin.net/atpiii/calculator.asp?usertype=prof.

- National Heart, Lung, and Blood Institute, National Cholesterol Education Program (NCEP). "Third Report of the Expert Panel on Detection, Evaluation, and Treatment of High Blood Cholesterol in Adults (ATP III Final Report)." http://www.nhlbi.nih.gov/guidelines/cholesterol/atp3_rpt.htm.

- Thyroid.org. http://www.thyroid.org/patients/brochures.html.

1 Which of Margie's lab values are outside the normal range?

_____

_____

2 What problem does Margie likely have?

_____

3 What is the cause of Margie's problem?

_____

_____

_____

_____

_____

_____

_____

4 What are the typical symptoms of Margie's problem?

_____

_____

_____

_____

_____

_____

_____

_____

5 How will Margie's problem be treated?

_____

_____

_____

_____

_____

6 What other disease can result from too-aggressive treatment of Margie's problem?

_____

_____

_____

_____

_____

_____

_____

_____

_____

_____

_____

_____

_____

_____

_____

_____

A Piercing Issue

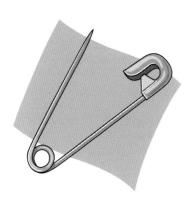

Jessica Gangly, a 17-year-old, has a doctor's appointment at 8 a.m. She reports that her heart is "doing funny things." She has been attending dance camp and says she is fine in the morning but starts to feel "strange" by about 11 a.m. "My heart seems to skip beats, and then it stops for what seems like five seconds. Then it pounds. Sometimes I get these really rapid heartbeats, and I see stars. My heart hurts, too—sort of a piercing pain. I'm doing dance camp because I want to model when I get out of high school. I'll never be a hand-and-foot model—I have man hands and flat feet—but I think I could do runway. Dance is helping me walk and move with some grace . . . um . . . which is sort of difficult at my height. I love clothes and design. Give me a few safety pins, and I can take just about any outfit and morph it into an edgy style."

Jessica is given a physical and an ECG. Selected results are given below:

- Height: 6'0" (183 cm)
- Weight: 120 lbs. (54.4 kg)
- BP: 110/67
- Temp: 38°C
- Lung auscultation: No abnormal findings
- Heart auscultation: No abnormal findings; no midsystolic click; no late systolic murmur
- ECG: Normal sinus rhythm
- ENT: Multiple conjunctival hemorrhages
- Wears contact lenses
- Teeth, palate not remarkable; last dental exam four months ago
- No lymphadenopathy
- Family history: Not remarkable; parents and both sets of grandparents are alive; no history of sudden cardiac death, stroke, other cardiovascular disease, diabetes, or cancer; no history of thoracic aortic aneurysm
- Patient is tall and thin with long fingers and long flat feet; wears contact lenses and reports that she has a "−6.50" prescription
- Patient complains of muscle aches, joint pain, and fatigue that she attributes to long hours of dancing at camp

Blood is drawn and sent to the lab. Jessica is scheduled at 11:30 a.m. for an echocardiogram, an ultrasound series of images of the heart obtained from the reflection or transmission of ultrasonic waves through cardiac (heart and aorta) tissue. After being asked if anyone in her family has ever been told that he or she has a thoracic aortic aneurysm, Jessica says she is beginning to feel very anxious. She says, "No one in my family—but a famous model dropped dead of it on the runway in Paris last year!"

Below is the report from her echocardiogram.

Echocardiography Laboratory

Name: Jessica Gangly

Age: 17

Findings

- **Indications:** History of palpitations
- **ECG rhythm:** Sinus rhythm with several PACs, PVCs
- **Study quality:** Transthoracic M-Mode, Two Dimensional, Pulsed Doppler, Color Doppler, and Continuous Wave Doppler were performed. The study was technically adequate.
- **Left ventricle global:** LV size, wall thickness, and systolic function are normal, with an EF > 60%
- **Right ventricle:** The right ventricle is mildly enlarged, measuring between 31 and 35 mm. The right ventricular systolic function is normal.
- **Left atrium:** The left atrium is normal in size.
- **Right atrium:** The right atrium is normal in size.
- **Aortic valve:** The aortic valve is trileaflet and appears structurally normal, with no aortic stenosis or regurgitation.
- **Mitral valve:** The mitral valve is thickened with myxomatus degeneration. There is trace mitral regurgitation. There is mild thickening of the posterior mitral valve leaflet and mild prolapse of the anterior mitral valve leaflet.
- **Tricuspid valve:** The tricuspid appears structurally normal. There is trace/mild (physiological) regurgitation.
- **Pulmonic valve:** Pulmonic valve appears structurally normal, physiological degree of pulmonic regurgitation.
- **Thrombus:** There was no evidence of intracardiac thrombus.
- **Aorta:** Limited views of the ascending aorta and the descending thoracic aorta are of normal caliber with no significant atherosclerotic disease or aneurysmal dilatation.
- **IVC:** The inferior vena cava is normal.
- **Pericardium:** The pericardium is normal, and there is no pericardial effusion.

Conclusions

- The left ventricle is normal in size and function with EF greater than 60%.
- There is no evidence of significant diastolic abnormality.
- The aortic root size is normal.
- There is no evidence of thoracic aortic dilation.
- The right ventricle is mildly dilated.
- There is no evidence of significant valve stenosis.
- There is mild MVP with trace MR noted.
- There is no pericardial effusion.

References

- American Heart Association. "Prophylaxis Guidelines." http://www.ada.org/2157.aspx.
- Autonomic and Mitral Valve Prolapse Disorder Center. http://www.mvprolapse.com.
- National Marfan Foundation. "Marfan Syndrome." http://www.marfan.org/marfan.
- Plewa, M. C. 2011. "Mitral Valve Prolapse." *eMedicine* (June 27). http://eMedicine.medscape.com/article/759004-overview.

1   What do a midsystolic click and late systolic murmur indicate?

_____

_____

_____

_____

_____

_____

_____

2   Why was an echocardiogram ordered if Jessica's physical exam was normal?

_____

_____

_____

_____

_____

_____

_____

_____

_____

_____

_____

_____

_____

_____

3   What is a thoracic aortic aneurysm? What are the risks? How can it be treated?

_____

_____

_____

_____

_____

4   What does Jessica's echocardiogram report show?

_____

_____

_____

_____

_____

_____

_____

_____

5   What can be done for Jessica's heart rhythm problem?

_____

_____

_____

_____

_____

_____

_____

6 When Jessica's serology comes back from the lab, she is called to return immediately for an appointment for another blood culture. Both blood cultures, drawn 12 hours apart, are positive for *Staphylococcus aureus*. She undergoes another type of echocardiogram called transesophageal echocardiography (TEE). In this procedure, the patient is subjected to conscious sedation with a drug such as propofol (the patient is awake but will have no memory of the procedure). A local anesthetic is sprayed in the throat. The patient then lies on the left side and swallows the ultrasound probe until it is positioned in the esophagus directly behind the heart. A screenshot of the TEE follows. What other problem does Jessica have, as shown on the transesophageal echocardiogram?

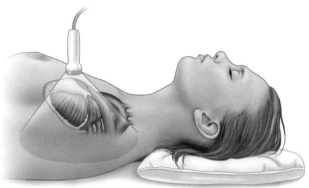

24-1 Standard or transthoracic echo

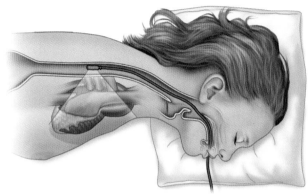

24-2 Transesophageal echo or TEE

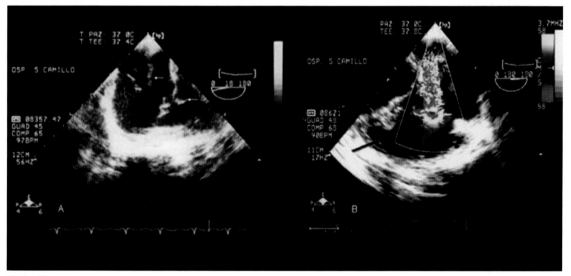

24-3 **Images from TEE procedure** The arrows on the image on the left (A) point to two bacterial vegetations on the eustachian and tricuspid valves. The image on the right shows color Doppler imaging detecting regurgitation from the tricuspid valve toward the eustachian valve.

Adriano M. Pellicelli, Paulo Pino, Antonio Terranova, Cecilia D'Ambrosio, and Fabrizio Soccorsi,
"Eustachian Valve Endocarditis: A Rare Localization of Right Side Endocarditis," Copyright 2005 Biomed Central, www.biomedcentral.com

7 What was the likely cause of this problem?

_____

_____

_____

_____

_____

_____

_____

_____

_____

_____

_____

_____

Kidney Punch

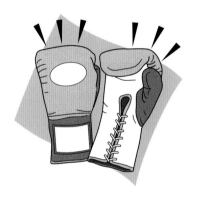

Gerry M., age 23, is an amateur boxer and lays carpet for a living. He states that he had a calcium oxalate kidney stone about three weeks ago and went to the emergency department because the pain was so bad. The stone passed while he was waiting for treatment. He felt fine after that and went back to his previous routine. Then, two weeks ago, his left elbow was sore, red, and swollen when he woke up in the morning. He went to the emergency department and was diagnosed with olecranon bursitis and given a prescription for ibuprofen (800 mg four times a day). Today he is back at the emergency department complaining of severe pain in his lower back (in the area of the costovertebral angle on both sides), and his bursitis has not resolved.

Bursal fluid is aspirated from his left elbow and analyzed.

He is given an axial CT scan of his lower abdomen, in which after a CT scan is taken, the table on which the patient is situated is moved a tiny bit, and another scan is taken. This process is called "step and shoot." The CT scan machine then uses tomographic reconstruction to generate a three-dimensional axial image.

Gerry M. goes into acute renal failure and is placed on the kidney/liver transplant list.

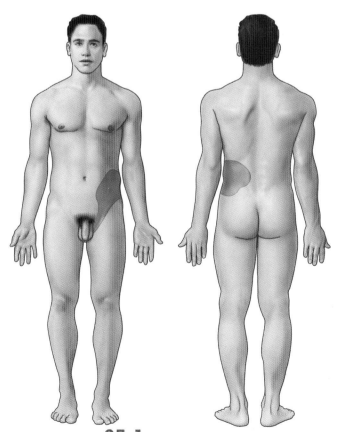

25-1 Region of pain

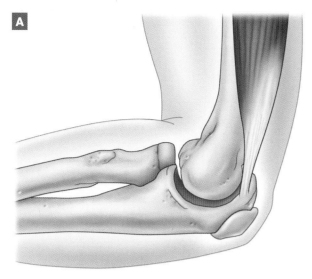

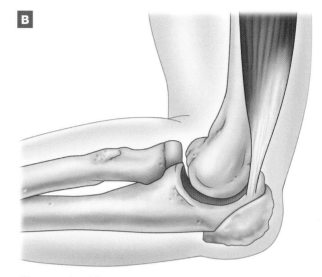

Olecranon bursa

Olecranon bursitis

25-2 (A) **Normal olecranon bursa and** (B) **olecranon bursitis**

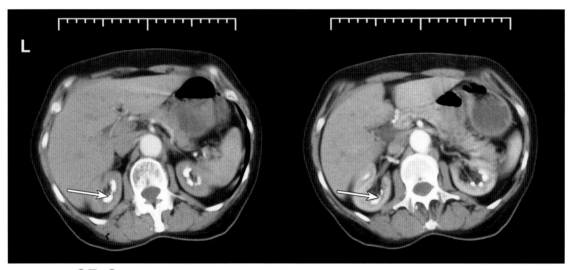

25-3 **Axial CT scan** Note calcium deposits in the medulla of both kidneys.

References

- Khan, A. N. 2011. "Nephrocalcinosis." *Medscape Reference.* http://emedicine.medscape.com/article/379449-overview#a20.

- National Foundation for Transplants. http://www.transplants.org.

- National Kidney Foundation. "Kidney Stones." http://www.kidney.org/atoz/atozTopic_KidneyStones.cfm.

- OrganDonor.gov. http://www.organdonor.gov.

- Oxalosis and Hyperoxaluria Foundation. http://www.ohf.org.

- U.S. Department of Health and Human Services, U.S. Government Information on Organ and Tissue Donation and Transplantation. http://www.organdonor.gov.

Questions

1 What are the symptoms of kidney stones (nephrolithiasis)?

2 What is the etiology of nephrolithiasis?

3 How can the risk of future episodes of nephrolithiasis be reduced?

4 What are the symptoms of olecranon bursitis?

5 What is the etiology of olecranon bursitis?

6 What do you expect will be found in the bursal fluid?

_____

_____

_____

_____

7 What is causing Gerry's lower back pain now?

_____

_____

_____

_____

_____

_____

_____

8 What are the risk factors for this current condition?

_____

_____

_____

_____

_____

_____

9 What are the treatments for this condition?

_____

_____

_____

_____

_____

_____

10 Why will Gerry M. need a kidney/liver transplant?

Night Watch

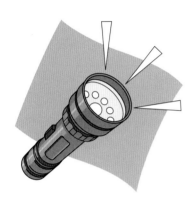

After Desmond Dow retired from the police force of a small midwestern city, he took a job as a night watchman for an insurance company. After 25 years of detective work, rounds on the 30-story building were, in a word, "boring." But he was determined to persevere for two more years until his wife could retire from her third-shift nursing supervisor's job. Much of Mr. Dow's shift involved watching monitors. His weight had crept upward. "At 275, I'd be in trouble if I were still on the force," he said.

As his weight increased, so did his indigestion. At first antacid tablets seemed to work—but then he realized that he was taking them every two hours. He started taking an acid reducer/antacid combination (Pepcid AC), and this seemed to work for a few months. Then he saw an ad on TV for a new over-the-counter acid reducer that promised 'round-the-clock acid reduction. He found a generic version of omeprazole (Prilosec OTC) in the corner store and took that for three months.

When he went for his annual physical, he reported "I'm tired all the time. I think it's just my late-shift work—I don't think it suits my biological clock. My other problem is my indigestion. Last Thursday I was eating a corn dog, and the thing seemed to get stuck in my esophagus. Wow, did I suffer that night! I've had a hiatal hernia all my life. I keep my head propped up with pillows at night, and I don't go to bed until at least three hours after eating. . . . Well, I used to do this anyway, until I took this night job."

Mr. Dow's only prescription drug is amlodipine (Norvasc), 10 mg per day for hypertension. His blood pressure was at target at his office visit: 135/80. Mr. Dow's fasting blood values are on the following page. He was also sent to a gastroenterologist, who performed an endoscopic exam. (See Grandma's Got a Brand-New Bag, Case 7, for a discussion of endoscopic upper GI exams.)

Below are the results of his lab tests.

Mr. Dow's Lab Results

Test	Value	SI Units	Reference Range	SI Units
Ammonia	47 mcg/dL	28 µmol/L	19–60 mcg/dL	11–35 µmol/L
BUN	12 mg/dL	4.3 mmol/L	7–18 mg/dL	2.5–6.9 mmol/L
Creatinine, serum	1.1 mg/dL	97 µmol/L	0.8–1.3 mg/dL	71–115 µmol/L
Bilirubin, total	0.7 mg/dL	12 µmol/L	0.1–1.0 mg/dL	1.7–17.1 µmol/L
Bilirubin, direct (conjugated)	0.1 mg/dL	1.7 µmol/L	0.1–0.3 mg/dL	1.7–5.1 µmol/L
Bilirubin, indirect (unconjugated)	0.4 mg/dL	6.8 µmol/L	0.2–0.8 mg/dL	3.4–13.7 µmol/L
Protein, total	7.5 g/dL	75 g/L	6.4–8.2 g/dL	64–82 g/L
Albumin	4.4 g/dL	44 g/L	3.4–5.0 g/dL	34–50 g/L
Alkaline phosphatase	125 U/L		50–136 U/L	
Aspartate aminotransferase (AST)	29 U/L		15–37 U/L	
Alanine amino-transferase (ALT)	51U/L		30–65 U/L	
Gamma-glutamyl transferase (GGT)	79 U/L		1–94 U/L	
Cholesterol, total	220 mg/dL	5.7 mmol/L	50–199 mg/dL	1.3–5.2 mmol/L
Triglycerides	149 mg/dL	1.7 mmol/L	15–149 mg/dL	0.17–1.7 mmol/L
LDL, direct	140 mg/dL	3.6 mmol/L	0–99 mg/dL	0.0–2.6 mmol/L
HDL	45 mg/dL	1.2 mmol/L	> 40 mg/dL	> 1 mmol/L
RBC	4.1 K/cmm		4.50–5.90 K/cmm	
Hemoglobin (HGB)	15.5 g/dL	155 g/L	13.5–17.5 g/dL	135–175 g/L
Hematocrit (HCT)	53.0%		41.0–53.0%	
Mean corpuscular volume (MCV)	105 fL		80–100 fL	
Mean corpuscular hemoglobin (MCH)	29 pg		26.0–34.0 pg	
Mean corpuscular hemoglobin concentration (MCHC)	32.0 g/dL	320 g/L	31.0–37.0 g/dL	310–370 g/L
Prothrombin time (PT)	10 seconds		9–12 seconds	

Below right is a photograph of an abnormal finding on endocsopic exam of Mr. Dow's esophagus. A biopsy was taken for further examination.

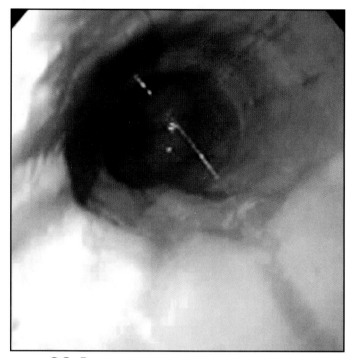

26-1 Normal endoscope of esophagus

26-2 Abnormal endoscope of esophagus

Courtesy of Medical College of Wisconsin

Below is a photomicrograph of the abnormal cells removed from Mr. Dow's esophagus.

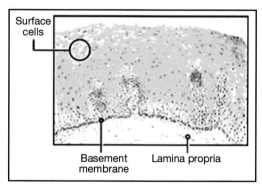

26-3 Photomicrograph of normal esophageal cells

Courtesy of Barrettsinfo.com

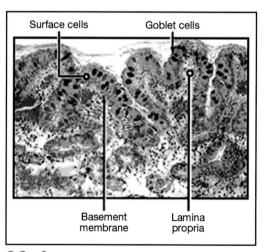

26-4 Photomicrograph of Mr. Dow's abnormal esophageal cells

Courtesy of Barrettsinfo.com

The biopsy revealed that the normal stratified squamous epithelium was replaced by metaplastic, specialized, columnar glandular epithelium known as "specialized intestinal metaplasia of the esophagus."

References

■ American College of Gastroenterology, Patient Education and Resource Center. "Barrett's Esophagus." http://patients.gi.org/topics/barretts-esophagus.

■ Buttar, N. S., and K. Wang. 2004. "Mechanisms of Disease: Carcinogenesis in Barrett's Esophagus." *Nature Clinical Practice Gastroenterology and Hepatology* (December 27). http://www.medscape.com/viewarticle/495345.

■ Institute of Medicine. 1998. "Dietary Reference Intakes for Thiamin, Riboflavin, Niacin, Vitamin B_{12}, Pantothenic Acid, Biotin, and Choline: A Report of the Standing Committee on the Scientific Evaluation of Dietary Reference Intakes and Its Panel on Folate, Other B Vitamins, and Choline/Subcommittee on Upper Reference Levels of Nutrients, Food and Nutrition Board, Institute of Medicine." Washington, DC: National Academy of Sciences. http://books.nap.edu/openbook.php?record_id=6015&page=306.

1 What do Mr. Dow's lab values suggest?

_____

_____

2 What are the possible causes of these abnormal lab values?

_____

_____

_____

_____

_____

_____

3 What other lab values do you think will be ordered to confirm your suspicions?

_____

_____

_____

4 What problems does Mr. Dow have with his esophagus? What does the biopsy suggest?

_____

_____

_____

_____

_____

_____

_____

_____

_____

5 What future problem is Mr. Dow now at risk for?

6 How will Mr. Dow be treated?

7 What lifestyle changes can help improve Mr. Dow's symptoms?

The Hoarse Horsewoman

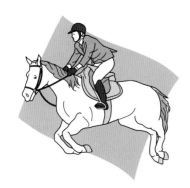

Brittany Shores is an accomplished equestrian who volunteers 20 hours per week teaching children with special needs how to ride and care for horses. She is in the Ear, Nose, and Throat Clinic today. She says, "By Wednesday, I have no voice. This has been going on for about four months now. Last Monday I woke up and literally couldn't speak. I have a chronic cough, too, but I've had that for years. It's from breathing hay. I usually wear a mask when I muck out the barn."

A physical exam and medical history reveals the following:

- Age: 51
- Height/weight: 5'4" (162.6 cm) 140 lbs. (63.5 kg) (has lost 15 lbs. [6.8 kg] in the past year)
- Blood pressure: 115/70
- Pulse: 64
- Former cigarette smoker (one pack a day from ages 18–28)
- Chronic cough produces scant sputum with blood streaks
- Adopted, no family history available

A chest X-ray is ordered and is shown below:

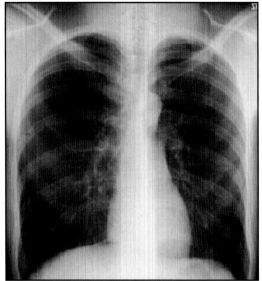

27-1 Normal X-ray

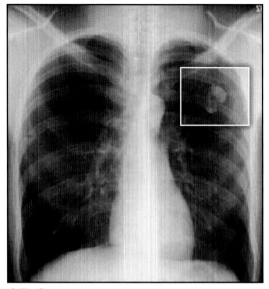

27-2 Brittany's X-ray

Following the X-ray, a spiral CT scan is ordered. A spiral CT scan is different from a regular CT scan in that the patient is moved rapidly through the spiral CT scanner. Spiral CT scans produce images with higher definition of blood vessels and internal tissues within the chest cavity. Images from the spiral CT scan are shown below.

(Note A is aorta, S is spine.)

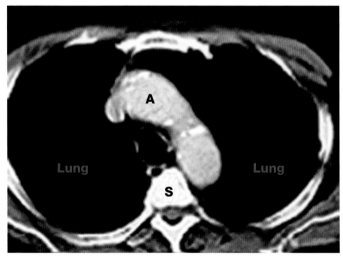

27-3 Normal spiral CT scan

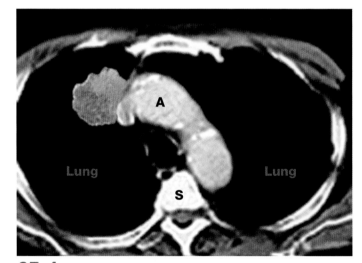

27-4 Brittany's spiral CT scan

References

- American Society of Clinical Oncology. 2012. "The Role of CT Screening for Lung Cancer in Clinical Practice." http://www.asco.org/ASCOv2/Practice+%26+Guidelines/Guidelines/Clinical+Practice+Guidelines.

- "Lung Cancer in Women." *Harvard Health*. http://www.health.harvard.edu/articles/lung_cancer.htm.

- Tan, W. W. 2012. "Small Cell Lung Cancer." *eMedicine* (December 27). http://eMedicine.medscape.com/article/280104-overview.

1 What underlying problem does Brittany Shores appear to have? What are the four major types of this problem?

_____

_____

_____

2 How common is this problem in women?

_____

_____

   a. How susceptible are women to this problem compared with men?

_____

_____

   b. How does the prognosis vary between men and women?

_____

_____

_____

_____

3 What are the possible causes of this problem?

_____

_____

_____

_____

_____

_____

_____

_____

_____

4   Why does this problem present as laryngitis? (Consider the anatomy of the laryngeal nerve in your answer.)

5   What are the screening tests for early diagnosis of this problem?

6   What are the clinical signs of this problem?

7   What are the treatment options for this problem?

The ATV Riders

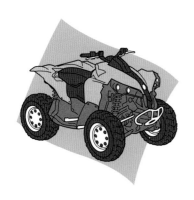

Cheryl and Sean enjoy riding their ATVs at night on the back roads under the full moon and stars. One night Cheryl bumped over a hole and fell off her ATV next to a stone wall. Sean could not avoid running over her and hitting the stone wall. He fell off his ATV, hit his head, and became unconscious. His ATV landed on Cheryl, crushing both of her legs. She was unable to reach her cellphone to call for help.

Nearly four hours later, Sean "came to" and was able to dial 911. He pulled the ATV off Cheryl. The LifeStar helicopter arrived within 15 minutes. "Wish you hadn't pulled the ATV off your wife yet," said the paramedic. "We wanted to hook her up to a cardiac monitor, give her albuterol via a nebulizer, and hook her up to a fluid IV before we relieved the crush."

"But she doesn't even have any bruises or swelling," Sean responded. "And she didn't have any pain until *after* I removed the ATV."

The paramedics did their work. They put in two IVs of normal saline at 500 ml/hour total. They also gave Cheryl a dose of sodium bicarbonate (in the IV bag) and fentanyl (an opioid) for pain. Then LifeStar transported both Cheryl and Sean to the nearest trauma center, a 15-minute chopper ride away.

Sean was diagnosed with a severe concussion. His vital signs and results of an MRI were within normal limits. He was admitted for observation.

Cheryl suffered crush injury syndrome, which results from a severe crush injury over an extensive portion of the body that lasts for a prolonged period, typically four to six hours of compression.

Following are serial ECGs—one taken immediately after the paramedics arrived and one five minutes later in the chopper.

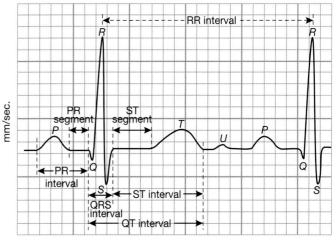

mm/mV   1 square = 0.04 sec/01.mV

28-1 Normal ECG

From the *Merck Manual of Diagnosis and Therapy*, 18th ed., edited by Mark H. Beers.

© 2006 by Merck & Co., Inc., Whitehouse Station, NJ. Available at www.merck.com.

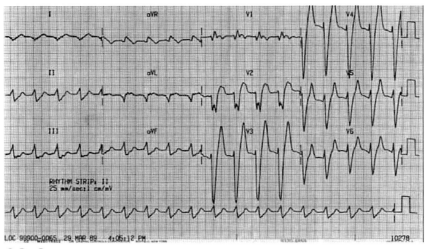

28-2 **Cheryl's initial ECG** Note widened QRS complexes, flat and wide P waves, ventricular ectopic beats; serum potassium is probably ~ 7.5–8.5 mEq/L.

Courtesy of www.emedicine.com, 2008

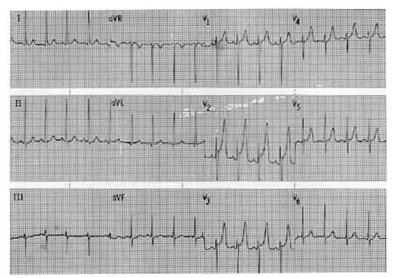

28-3 **Cheryl's ECG 5 minutes after IV of normal saline and dose of sodium bicarbonate** Note improvement: QRS less wide; there are peaked T waves; serum potassium is ~ 5.5–6.5 mEq/L.

Courtesy of www.emedicine.com, 2008

When Cheryl arrived at the trauma center, her hands were in an unusual position:

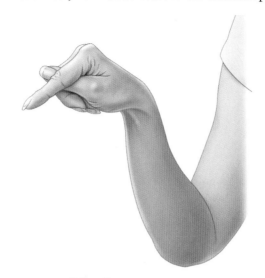

28-4 Cheryl's hand

Her ECG follows:

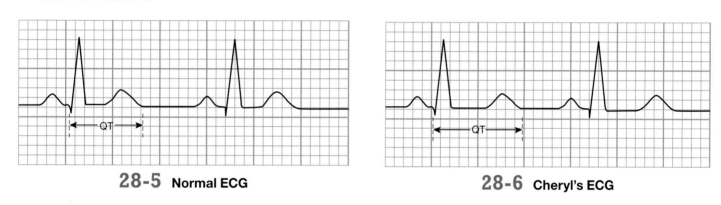

28-5 Normal ECG

28-6 Cheryl's ECG

Cheryl had a Foley catheter inserted, and mannitol was added to her IV infusion to maintain urine output. Her urine had a dark, red-brown color. She was given an infusion of glucose and insulin.

Below are selected lab values for Cheryl five minutes later.

Test	Value	SI Units	Reference Range (non-fasting)	SI Units
Glucose	115 mg/dL	6.4 mmol/L	< 200 mg/dL	< 11.1 mmol/L
BUN	18 mg/dL	6.4 mmol/L	7–18 mg/dL	2.5–6.4 mmol/L
Creatinine, serum	1.9 mg/dL	168 µmol/L	0.8–1.3 mg/dL	71–115 µmol/L
Bilirubin, total	1.2 mg/dL	20.5 µmol/L	0.1–1.0 mg/dL	1.71–17.1 µmol/L
Protein, total	6.5 g/dL	75 g/L	6.4–8.2 g/dL	64–82 g/L
Albumin	3.4 g/dL	44 g/L	3.4–5.0 g/dL	34–50 g/L
Creatine phosphokinase (CK)	80,000 IU/L		8–150 IU/L	
WBC	5.1 K/cmm		4.5–11.0 K/cmm	
RBC	4.0 K/cmm		4.00–5.20 K/cmm	
HGB	11.9 g/dL	119 g/L	12.0–16.0 g/dL	120–160 g/L
HCT	35.8%		36.0–46.0%	
MCV	90 fL		80–100 fL	
MCH	31.2 pg		26.0–34.0 pg	
MCHC	33.7 g/dL	337 g/L	31.0–37.0 g/dL	310–370 g/L
Sodium	140 mEq/L	140 mmol/L	136–145 mEq/L	136–145 mmol/L
Potassium	5.5 mEq/L	5.5 mmol/L	3.5–5.1 mEq/L	3.5–5.1 mmol/L
Chloride	108 mEq/L	108 mmol/L	98–107 mEq/L	98–107 mmol/L
Calcium	8.0 mg/dL	2 mmol/L	8.5–10.5 mg/dL	2.1–2.6 mmol/L
Phosphorus	4.9 mg/dL	1.58 mmol/L	3–4.5 mg/dL	0.8–1.4 mmol/L

One of Cheryl's IV lines was removed and carefully flushed with sterile water. Then Cheryl was given calcium chloride by slow IV push (over a period of 60 seconds).

References

- Garth, D. 2012. "Hyperkalemia." *eMedicine* (April 25). http://www.eMedicine.com/emerg/topic261.htm.

- Krost, W. S., J. J. Mistovich, and D. Limmer. 2008. "Beyond the Basics: Crush Injuries and Compartment Syndrome." *Emergency Medical Services*. http://www.emsresponder.com/print/Emergency--Medical-Services/Beyond-the-Basics--Crush-Injuries-and-Compartment-Syndrome/1$7056.

- Pegoraro, A. A., and G. W. Rutecki. 2011. "Hypocalcemia." *eMedicine* (October 27). http://www.eMedicine.com/med/topic1118.htm.

- Vanholder, R., A. van der Tol, M. De Smet, E. Hoste, M. Koc, A. Hussain, S. Khan, and M. S. Sever. 2007. "Earthquakes and Crush Syndrome Casualties: Lessons Learned from the Kashmir Disaster." *Kidney International* 71: 17–23. http://www.nature.com/ki/journal/v71/n1/full/5001956a.html.

Questions

1 Why did the paramedic state that the cardiac monitor, IV fluid line, and albuterol should be administered *before* removing the quad?

_____

_____

_____

2 Albuterol is a bronchodilator. What is released in crush injury syndrome that would cause bronchoconstriction?

_____

_____

3 What toxic substances released from crushed muscle can affect the heart? (*Hint:* Consider two different minerals released from crushed muscle.)

_____

_____

_____

_____

4 What toxic substances released from crushed muscle can affect the kidneys?

_____

_____

5 The paramedics put in two IV lines of normal saline to counteract the expected hypovolemia and prevent hypovolemic shock. Why did they also administer sodium bicarbonate?

_____

_____

_____

_____

6 How can IV glucose and insulin correct hyperkalemia?

7 What do Cheryl's ECG, cramped hand, and lab values upon arrival at the trauma center suggest?

8 Why can't calcium chloride be put in the same infusion with sodium bicarbonate?

Index